Inner Transformation:
The Art and Science of Hypnosis

I0426971

Using the power of the subconscious mind
to transform lives.

Tim Moore
MHt, CHt, MNLP

Copyright 2024 Tim Moore

All rights reserved

For more information or to begin your journey as a professional hypnotherapist, visit

www.hypno-mastery.com

HYPNO-MASTERY

HYPNOTHERAPY TRAINING & CERTIFICATION

For individual private sessions and support, contact:
Mind Over The Body

www.mindoverthebody.com

1304 S. College Ave.
Fort Collins, Colorado, 80524

"Inner Transformation: The Art and Science of Hypnosis"

HYPNO-MASTERY

HYPNOTHERAPY TRAINING & CERTIFICATION

www.hypno-mastery.com

Your Inner Transformation!

I've seen and been part of some pretty amazing transformations by helping people use the power of their minds to create rapid change in their lives. Everything from fears, phobias, anxiety, depression, and pain, as they melt away quickly and easily. Some of my clients, despite seeing traditional counselors or therapists for years have been able to finally release the things that have been holding them back and bothering them in only a few sessions. This power is truly remarkable and resides within us all. The power to make subconscious changes can literally change someone's life in minutes.

This book is for those who want to explore learning these methods to help others, as well as those wanting to learn these tools for their own self-improvement. Whatever your reason for being here, you are going to gain some valuable tools for making permanent subconscious changes.

We will explore a number of different techniques including blending hypnosis with Neuro Linguistic Programming, Eye Movement Integration, Emotional Freedom techniques, and more.

Hypnosis can be one of the most powerful things you can do to improve nearly any aspect of life, but it's often a very misunderstood topic. At its core, hypnosis is a state of focused attention, heightened suggestibility, and vivid imagination. It's like being absorbed in a good book or movie; the outside world fades away, and you become engrossed in the narrative. You may have been so absorbed by that book that you start feeling emotions and physical sensations from those pages and stories. It certainly wasn't the black ink on the white paper that created those emotions and sensations, it was the amazing power of your subconscious mind. You allowed yourself to go into a trance state, focusing on creating the scenes in your mind, and your subconscious obeyed and took that story and made it feel real. This is very similar to the hypnotic state, and in that state, you can make some amazing life changes. Changes in fears, weight loss, overcoming bad habits, confidence, pain, and disease management, and just about any other human experience you can think of.

Contrary to what some may believe, hypnosis is not a state of sleep, and people under hypnosis are not unconscious. They are fully aware of what's happening, hear every word, and can't be made to do anything against their will. While Hollywood may make it seem like some mystical mind control, it's far from it. It is however your secret doorway into permanent subconscious change for life improvement though.

In this book, we will explore the therapeutic use of hypnosis for improving our lives and the lives of others (should you wish to explore using hypnosis professionally)

Hypnotherapy is the practice of using hypnosis as a tool to help overcome various psychological and physical conditions rather than something used for entertainment. A trained hypnotherapist, or you through self-hypnosis, can guide you to a resourceful state where permanent change can occur. A state of peace, relaxation, and calm, and once in this state, the mind is more open to positive suggestions and exploring new ideas and perspectives.

So how exactly does hypnotherapy work?

During a hypnotherapy session, the person hypnotized is not asleep or unconscious. They remain aware of their surroundings but are more open to suggestions. The hypnotherapist may use various techniques, such as

1.) Direct Suggestion: Utilizing the heightened suggestibility to encourage positive behavioral or cognitive changes. This can be effective for habits like smoking/vaping cessation or weight loss.
2.) Analytical Hypnotherapy: Also known as hypnoanalysis, this technique aims to resolve underlying psychological problems contributing to an unwanted lie condition or experience. It's often used for deeper issues like anxiety, depression, or phobias, removing pain or treatment side effects, and overcoming limiting beliefs while boosting confidence.

Hypnotherapy can be used for a wide range of issues, including:

- Stress and Anxiety Reduction: Helping individuals to relax and manage stress more effectively.
- Pain Management: Particularly for chronic pain or pain associated with medical procedures.
- Disease management to overcome treatment side effects.
- Overcoming Bad Habits: Like smoking or vaping (or any unwanted habits)
- Addictions
- Improving Sleep: Helping with issues like insomnia.
- Weight Loss without supplements or strict diets
- Enhancing Performance: Useful in sports psychology or public speaking.
- Overcoming self-doubt and limiting beliefs.

Hypnotherapy is completely safe for most people when conducted by a trained and qualified professional. However, it's not suitable for everyone. People with severe mental health issues or those prone to psychotic episodes, such as hallucinations or delusions, should consult a medical professional before considering hypnotherapy.

Hypnosis should also not be used as a replacement for medical or mental health care by a licensed practitioner. Hypnosis is a powerful complementary therapy that can greatly improve outcomes. The end results are ultimately up to the person being hypnotized.

Hypnosis and hypnotherapy are intriguing fields that blend psychology and the power of suggestion. With a trained therapist, hypnotherapy can be a valuable tool for personal development and healing. Remember, it's about guidance and suggestion, not control. The power of hypnotherapy is in its ability to tap into the subconscious mind, promoting positive change and self-improvement.

The goal of this book is to fulfill a threefold purpose: to educate, demystify, and provide practical guidance in the use of hypnosis. Each of these aspects is extremely important in delivering a complete understanding of what hypnosis and hypnotherapy are, and how you can use it to create positive change for yourself or others.

Educate: The primary goal of the book is to impart knowledge. This involves presenting information in a clear, understandable manner that is accessible to a wide range of readers, regardless of your prior knowledge of hypnosis. The book will cover fundamental concepts, theories, and historical perspectives, providing a solid foundation for those interested in improving their own lives, or those wishing to explore hypnotherapy professionally. The goal of this book is to give you the resources to not only learn about hypnosis and the power of the subconscious mind but also understand its relevance and application in the real world.

Demystify: A key objective is to dispel myths and misconceptions surrounding the topic of hypnosis. Many subjects, especially those like hypnotherapy or other specialized fields, are often shrouded in mystery and misinformation. My goal is to clarify these misunderstandings by presenting facts and evidence-based information. This involves tackling common myths head-on, explaining why they are false, and replacing them with accurate information. By doing so, we can help break down barriers of skepticism and fear, making hypnosis more approachable and less intimidating.

Provide Practical Guidance: Beyond theoretical knowledge, I intend to offer practical advice and strategies that you can apply in everyday life. The purpose of this book is to create a comprehensive resource that not only imparts knowledge and corrects misconceptions but also serves as a practical guide for you to apply what you have learned in a meaningful way. This approach ensures that this book is not only informative but also empowering, enabling you to gain a deeper understanding of hypnosis and how it can be applied to your life.

Now let's dive into this amazing resource and make some subconscious shifts!

Chapter 1

The History of Hypnosis.

In order to demystify the art of hypnosis, it's important to look at how trance states and suggestions evolved over time. While many see hypnosis as some form of entertainment or far-out concept, the reality is that some form of hypnosis or trance has been used throughout history. It seems that only in modern times we've forgotten that often times the fastest way to positive change is often the simplest. What could be easier than directing your mind and putting it on the path to change, and getting the conscious and subconscious mind in alignment?

Ancient and Medieval Period

- Shamanistic Rituals: In tribal societies, shamans used altered states of consciousness for healing and spiritual purposes. These states, often induced through repetitive drumming, dancing, and chanting, bear a resemblance to hypnotic trance states.
- Sleep Temples of Egypt: These temples, dating back to the second millennium BC, were centers for healing where priests used hypnotic techniques, possibly involving incantations and dream interpretation, to treat various ailments.
- Greek Healing Temples: In ancient Greece, temples dedicated to the god Asclepius practiced forms of healing that involved inducing dream states, which were considered divine messages offering guidance for healing.

17th and 18th Century – The Early Pioneers

- Paracelsus: This Swiss physician was a pioneer in the use of magnets for healing. While his methods were not hypnosis per se, they influenced later practitioners like Mesmer in the exploration of 'animal magnetism'.
- Franz Anton Mesmer: Mesmer developed a theory of 'animal magnetism' and used magnets and later his hands to manipulate what he believed were magnetic fluids in the body. His dramatic public demonstrations laid the foundation for later developments in hypnotism, despite being discredited by a scientific commission that included Benjamin Franklin.
- Marquis de Puységur: He discovered that a patient could enter a trance without Mesmer's theatrics, simply through calming techniques and suggestions. This was a significant move towards modern hypnotherapy.

19th Century – The Era of Refinement

- James Braid: Braid observed that focusing attention on a single object could lead to a trance-like state (think of the stereotypical swinging pocket watch). He initially thought this state was a form of sleep, but later realized it was a focused state of attention and coined the term 'hypnosis'. ("Hypno" is the word for sleep in ancient Greek)
- Ambroise-Auguste Liébeault and Hippolyte Bernheim: These French practitioners focused on the power of suggestion in the hypnotic state, moving the practice further away from Mesmer's magnetism theory.
- Jean-Martin Charcot: He primarily used hypnosis to treat hysteria and neurological disorders. Charcot's work was influential in legitimizing hypnosis in medical circles but was later critiqued for its focus on pathology.

- Sigmund Freud: Initially interested in hypnosis, Freud used it to explore the unconscious mind. Although he later abandoned hypnosis for psychoanalysis, his early work contributed significantly to the understanding of the psychological aspects of hypnosis. Freud saw the subconscious as a deep dark place, instead of the resourceful place to make changes that we recognize today.

20th Century – Further Refinement and Acceptance

- World Wars I & II: Hypnosis was used as a means of treating shell shock (now known as PTSD) in soldiers. Notably, during World Wars I and II, it was also used as an anesthetic for surgeries when chemical anesthesia was unavailable or impractical. Reports from these times suggest that hypnosis was effective in reducing pain and anxiety in many cases, and actually had higher success in surgical outcomes than surgeries done with chemical anesthesia.
- Milton H. Erickson: Erickson's approach was characterized by flexibility and non-directive techniques. He used storytelling, metaphors, and indirect suggestions to induce trance and facilitate change. (more on Erickson later)
- Clinical Recognition: The American Medical Association, no longer able to deny the powerful successes in treatment outcomes, finally recognized hypnotherapy in 1958, legitimizing it as a therapeutic practice. This recognition was a significant milestone in the integration

of hypnosis into mainstream medical and psychological practices.
- Dave Elman: Elman's methods, particularly his rapid induction techniques, were influential in the field of hypnosis. He emphasized the practical and clinical aspects of hypnosis, especially in pain control.

21st Century – Integration and Innovation

- Cognitive-Behavioral Hypnotherapy: This approach combines hypnotherapy with cognitive-behavioral techniques, providing a more holistic approach to treating disorders like anxiety, phobias, and stress.
- Evidence-Based Research: The increasing focus on evidence-based practice in medicine and psychology has led to more rigorous research on the efficacy of hypnosis, validating its use in various clinical settings.

The Future of Hypnotherapy

- Personalized Medicine: The trend towards personalized medicine may see hypnotherapy increasingly tailored to individual needs, based on genetic, lifestyle, and psychological profiles.
- Neuroscientific Research: Ongoing research in neuroscience is expected to shed light on how hypnosis affects different brain regions, potentially leading to new applications and techniques.

In modern hypnotherapy, two names stand out as having the greatest impact on hypnosis and hypnotherapy in today's age. Milton Erickson, possibly the greatest hypnotherapist to ever live, and Dave Elman who helped develop rapid induction techniques and showed how effective hypnosis is when combined with traditional healthcare.

Milton H. Erickson (1901–1980)

- Early Life: Erickson was born in 1901 in Nevada. Overcoming several personal challenges, including bouts of polio and color blindness, Erickson demonstrated early in life a deep interest in human psychology. When stricken with polio, Erickson became completely paralyzed. **While paralyzed and bed-ridden, Erickson developed phenomenal observation skills, to master verbal and non-verbal communication.**
- Education: He studied at the University of Wisconsin, receiving degrees in psychology and medicine. It was during his college years that he began to explore the field of hypnosis.
- Erickson's own experiences with polio, including a remarkable self-healing episode where he regained the ability to walk, greatly influenced his understanding of the mind-body connection and the potential of hypnosis.
- Innovative Techniques: Unlike traditional hypnotherapists of his time, Erickson used a more conversational, indirect approach to induce trance. He often employed storytelling, metaphors, and symbolism to engage the subconscious mind.

- Tailored Approach: Erickson believed that each individual was unique and required a customized approach. This led him to develop techniques that were adaptable to the specific needs and psychological makeup of each client.
- Teaching and Influence: Erickson was a prolific teacher and writer. His work greatly influenced the field of psychotherapy, particularly the development of strategic therapy, family systems therapy, and neuro-linguistic programming (NLP).
- Legacy: The Milton H. Erickson Foundation, established in 1979, continues to promote his teachings. Erickson's techniques remain widely used in hypnotherapy and psychotherapy, known for their efficacy in treating a range of psychological issues.

Dave Elman (1900–1967)

- Early Life and Career: Born in 1900, Elman had a varied career before delving into hypnosis. He initially worked in show business, including as a writer and composer for radio shows.
- Introduction to Hypnosis: Elman's interest in hypnosis was sparked by his father's experience with pain relief through hypnosis during a terminal illness. This personal connection deeply influenced his pursuit of hypnotherapy.
- Contributions to Hypnotherapy: Elman is best known for his development of rapid induction techniques. His method, often called the "Elman Induction," is famous for its efficiency and effectiveness in quickly inducing a deep hypnotic state.
- Focus on Medical Hypnosis: Elman's primary focus was on the medical applications of hypnosis, particularly in

pain management and anesthesia. He trained many physicians and dentists in his techniques, emphasizing the practical and clinical uses of hypnosis.

- Teaching and Lectures: Elman was a sought-after lecturer and teacher. His book "Hypnotherapy," published in 1964, remains a fundamental text in the field and is notable for its practical approach and clear, concise instructions.
- Legacy: Dave Elman's influence extends beyond traditional hypnotherapy; his techniques are used in various fields, including psychotherapy, dentistry, and emergency medicine. His emphasis on the practical application of hypnosis for pain control and medical procedures has left a lasting impact on the field.

Both Milton H. Erickson and Dave Elman revolutionized the field of hypnotherapy, each in their own unique way. Erickson's indirect and tailored approach expanded the psychological understanding and application of hypnosis, while Elman's rapid induction techniques and focus on medical hypnotherapy provided a practical framework for clinicians. Their legacies continue to influence modern therapeutic practices, illustrating the versatility and depth of hypnotherapy as a tool for healing and psychological change.

Chapter 2:

Understanding the Human Mind

Let's take a look into the human mind, the engine behind hypnosis and NLP. It's like unlocking a secret door to understand how our thoughts and feelings work. We'll explore the nitty-gritty of neuroscience and the relationship between what we're aware of (conscious mind) and what's running behind the scenes (subconscious mind).

If you imagine yourself as a computer, your body would be nothing more than the hardware, a pile of metal and plastic, unable to do anything when the operating system isn't running. The body has no ability to make any decisions. It's the operating system (your mind) that makes all of the decisions and controls all of the hardware and how it functions.

But here's the thing. That operating system needs a programmer to instruct it on what to tell the hardware to do. You have been programming that operating system your entire life through your past experiences. Sometimes throughout life, we let false information come into the subconscious and the operating system has a glitch that needs to be reprogrammed. Through hypnosis and NLP, you become that programmer. You can change a few lines of code and completely transform how that operating system performs.

Brain and Hypnosis – Like a Remote Control

- How the Brain Tunes In: Think of your brain as a high-tech control center. When hypnosis comes into play, it's like pressing specific buttons to change the channels of your thoughts. We'll look at how hypnosis can reroute pathways in your mind, making it a powerful tool for change.

- Brain Chemicals on a Joyride: Neurotransmitters are like tiny messengers sent from your body to the mind, and the reverse as well, and it's through hypnosis that we can direct how they deliver their messages, or what the response is to those signals.
- Your Inner Autopilot: Ever wonder why your heart beats faster when you're nervous? That's your autonomic nervous system at work, and your nervous system is under the complete control of the mind. Hypnosis can tap into this system, helping to calm your nerves or rev them up, depending on what's needed. Your mind is quite literally in control of everything, always working behind the scenes to regulate your blood pressure, tear production, body temperature, cell production, digestion, and every other function of your body. It's the great and powerful Oz behind the curtain.

The Conscious Mind – The Goal Setter

The conscious mind is like the CEO of a company. It's the part of you that makes decisions, thinks logically, and analyzes things coming in through your senses. In hypnosis, we need to work with this 'CEO' to get the green light for change. After getting that cooperation, we just need this CEO to step out of our way for a little bit so that we can have direct rapport with the subconscious mind without the boss's critical thinking getting in the way of making some changes.

The conscious mind also has a powerful accomplice. That's the critical factor. It's like the bouncer standing at the entry to the subconscious mind deciding what gets in and what doesn't. Our goal in hypnosis is to sneak past this bouncer and slip into the subconscious where change can be made.

The Subconscious Mind – Your Inner Genie in the Bottle

Your subconscious is where every one of your memories, habits, and deep-seated beliefs are stored. It's like a wizard with all the magic spells (memories and habits) tucked away in a secret filing cabinet. While we can't consciously recall everything stored in our subconscious, it has recorded every experience of our lives. Many of our beliefs, values, habits, and parts of our identity were given to us early in life by others before we had an opportunity to decide if those beliefs fit our worldview and aligned with our "I am" statement. We can however make changes that will transform our "I am" statement into the one we want.

Some people refer also to a third mind, the unconscious mind, but unconsciousness implies a state of not being aware or working. There is no unconsciousness in the way the conscious or subconscious works. It's on duty every second of your existence working in the background. Things that seem to be automatic like your heart beating, are things that we don't have to be consciously aware of, but you can be sure that the subconscious is fully aware and regulating it.

During hypnosis, we get to talk directly to this Genie in the bottle where once released, our wish is its command. It's like having a direct line to change habits or beliefs that you want to work on changing or improving.

The subconscious mind doesn't think, behave, or react at all like the conscious mind. When you hear self-talk in your mind (auditory digital), those thoughts are coming from your conscious mind. The conscious mind is the source of willpower, but imagination will always win over willpower. We want to use that willpower in alignment with our subconscious intention and to have the conscious and subconscious on the same team, with the same goals.

Think of your subconscious mind as a creative artist who doesn't speak much but loves showing you pictures, and movies, making you feel things, and using symbols or metaphors. Instead of telling you stuff straight up, it gives you these vivid dreams or those gut feelings that seem to pop up out of nowhere. It's always working in the background, putting together all your memories and feelings, and then communicating with you in its own artsy, emotional language. This is why when you're trying to understand your deeper self or sort out your feelings, it's not always about logic; it's more about tuning into these images and emotions that your subconscious is throwing your way.

It lives in its own world where reality and imagination blend together. Think about how when you daydream or imagine things vividly, it can feel real. That's your subconscious not really getting the difference between what's actually happening and what's in your head. And time? It doesn't care about that either. Things from way back when can feel just as important as what happened today in the realm of the subconscious.

Your subconscious also has its own moral code. It's got these deep beliefs and values that it sticks to, guiding how you act and react, often without you even realizing it. It's always there, kind of pulling the strings on your emotions and decisions. Understanding this part of your mind can be a game changer, giving you insights into why you do the things you do.

The Teamwork – Conscious and Subconscious Minds

Your conscious and subconscious minds don't always talk to each other, and sometimes they are out of alignment, but they influence each other more than you think. We'll explore how this teamwork is key in making lasting changes through hypnosis and NLP.

The power is in getting these 2 minds on the same team, working for the same outcome. We do that by giving direct suggestions. Think of a hypnotist as a skilled negotiator, finding ways to sneak good ideas past the conscious mind's defenses and into the subconscious. It's a bit like planting seeds in a garden – with time, they grow and flourish. The smallest seed can grow the tallest, strongest tree if the conditions are right.

Why This Matters – Real-World Hypnosis

Through hypnosis and NLP we are changing lives, one thought at a time: Understanding the brain's role in hypnosis isn't just cool science – it's a game-changer in therapy. We'll see how this knowledge can help in real-life situations, from overcoming fears, relieving pain, boosting self-esteem, building confidence, and a lot more.

This power isn't just for therapists or practitioners. Knowing about your mind's power can help you practice self-hypnosis and mindfulness, giving you tools to tweak your own thoughts, behaviors, emotions, and feelings.

Understanding the conscious and subconscious mind is like having a roadmap for the brain. It's crucial for anyone diving into the world of hypnosis – whether you're a pro or just curious about how your own mind works.

Chapter 3:
Principles of Hypnosis

Hypnosis and NLP (Neuro-Linguistic Programming) share common principles, but they also have unique aspects. Hypnosis focuses on guiding someone into a trance-like state to access the subconscious mind. It's about creating a deep state of relaxation and suggestibility to help change behaviors or thoughts.

NLP, on the other hand, is more about the connection between our language, thinking patterns, and behaviors. It's about understanding how we communicate with ourselves and others and using this insight to influence thoughts and behaviors in a positive way. NLP is about using both the conscious and subconscious to make change.

Both hypnosis and NLP are used to change unhelpful patterns and promote healthier, more positive ways of thinking and acting. They're about tapping into the power of the mind to make lasting changes. By combining these modalities we can some pretty remarkable changes in our lives.

The Science Behind The Trance

Hypnosis and Neuro-Linguistic Programming (NLP) are equally as fascinating in how they interact with the mind. When someone is hypnotized, it's not like they're asleep or unconscious. Instead, their brain activity changes in a way that makes them more open to suggestions and new ways of thinking. Research using EEGs has shown that during hypnosis, there's a shift in brain activity. This shift can lead to an altered state of consciousness, where the person is still aware but more focused internally, and less reactive to external stimuli. It's like the brain tunes into a different frequency, which can be really effective for therapy and personal development.

There are 5 brain wave frequencies that we can be in.

Gamma Waves (30-100 Hz): These are involved in higher mental activity and consolidation of information. When you're actively engaged in solving a complex problem, or deeply focused on a task, your brain is likely producing gamma waves.

Beta Waves (13-30 Hz): This your typical waking consciousness waves. When we are simply going about our day, we will generally be in low beta waves, but when we are fearful, anxious, or scared, we go into high beta. The fight, flight, or freeze response is linked to our brain's reaction to perceived threats or stress. During these states, our brain wave activity changes significantly. Typically, we go into high Beta waves, which are associated with alertness and decision-making. This heightened Beta activity helps us to quickly assess and respond to threats. In some cases, particularly during the freeze response, there might be a mix of Beta and Theta wave activity, reflecting a state of heightened alertness combined with a sort of mental paralysis. This complex interplay of brain waves under stress underscores how our brains rapidly adapt to ensure survival in threatening situations.

Alpha Waves (8-13 Hz): Alpha waves indicate a state of relaxed mental awareness or reflection. They're prevalent when you're daydreaming, practicing mindfulness, or in a light meditative state. They can also indicate a state of physical and mental relaxation while still being somewhat alert. Alpha frequency is generally where we will be most of the time during self-hypnosis and even some guided hypnosis. For change work such as weight loss or breaking habits, a light alpha state is usually all that is needed during trance.

Theta Waves (4-8 Hz): These occur in sleep and deep meditation. Theta waves are linked to creativity, intuition, daydreaming, and fantasizing. They represent the bridge to the subconscious and are associated with deeper emotional experiences. During hypnosis or a trance, your brain often slips into the Theta wave state, which is always my goal. Think of Theta waves like the state you're in just before you fall asleep or when you're daydreaming. They're all about deep relaxation and are key for hypnosis because they help you tap into your subconscious on a deeper level. This is where a lot of your deeper thoughts and feelings are stored. So, in this Theta state, you're more open to exploring and modifying these deep-seated beliefs and memories, making it a powerful tool for personal growth and understanding.

Delta Waves (0.5-4 Hz): These are the slowest and are found in deep, dreamless sleep or in very deep states of meditation. Delta waves are crucial for healing and regeneration. They are linked with deep unconsciousness and restorative sleep.

Each of these brain wave states reflects a different kind of processing in the brain, from high-alert problem-solving to deep, restful sleep.

People can sometimes resist going into hypnosis. First, the word "trance" itself might create resistance, even though trance is a natural state that we enter into several times a day. Another reason might be fear or a misunderstanding about what hypnosis is, or worry about losing control or being manipulated. Others may have skepticism about its effectiveness or have misconceptions based on how hypnosis is often portrayed in media. Personal discomfort with being in a vulnerable state or revealing hidden parts of the deeper self can also be a factor. It could also be as simple as having difficulty relaxing or letting go of conscious control. It's important for a hypnotherapist to address these concerns and build a trusting, comfortable environment for the process.

Crafting the Hypnotic Experience – Tools and Techniques

- Suggestion – The Heart of Hypnosis: We'll break down how suggestions work. It's like programming a computer; the hypnotist inputs suggestions and the client's subconscious mind runs the code.
- Imagery – Painting with Words: Here, we explore the power of mental imagery. Hypnotists use descriptive language to create vivid, sensory experiences in the client's mind, enhancing the depth of the hypnotic experience.
- Voice and Rhythm – The Hypnotist's Instruments: The hypnotist's voice is a powerful tool. We'll discuss how tone, pace, and rhythm can be used to guide someone into a trance and how these elements are as crucial as the words themselves.

The Client's Role – More Than Just a Participation

With hypnotherapy, the client plays a crucial role. It's not just about lying back and letting the therapist do all the work. Instead, the client needs to actively engage with the process. This means being open to the experience, willing to explore their thoughts and emotions, and actively participating in the session conversation. It's also about trust – trusting the therapist and the process. Clients need to be ready to embrace change and be honest with themselves, which can sometimes be challenging but is essential for effective change.

The reality is that all hypnosis is ultimately self-hypnosis. The hypnotic state is a self-generated state of focused, internal concentration. The hypnotist or hypnotherapist merely guides or facilitates the process, but the real change work is done by the individuals themselves. It's about using your own mind's ability to enter a state where change can happen more easily. This concept empowers people, emphasizing that they are in control and active participants in their own improvement.

The Critical Factor in Hypnosis: The Gatekeeper of the Mind

In the world of hypnosis, the "critical factor" is the door to change. Think of it like a mental gatekeeper or a personal bouncer for your thoughts and beliefs. It's part of your conscious mind and plays a crucial role in how we process information and accept or reject new ideas. The critical factor evaluates, judges, and analyzes incoming information based on our existing beliefs and experiences. It's like a filter that decides what gets into our subconscious mind.

Role of the Critical Factor in Hypnosis:

- In hypnosis, the goal is always to bypass this critical factor. Why? Because the critical factor can be a bit of a stickler for old rules and might block suggestions that could be beneficial in creating the changes we want. By bypassing it, a hypnotist can communicate directly with the subconscious mind, which is more open to accepting new ideas and suggestions since its job is to follow our commands.
- Good hypnotists don't just smash through this gate however; they gently and skillfully create an opening to slip through. Techniques like relaxation, focused attention, and the use of metaphors or stories are employed to ease the critical factor into a state where it's less vigilant and allows that door to be opened.

When someone's really analytical or skeptical, their mind's like a super alert guard, always questioning things. This doesn't mean they can't be hypnotized, but it does mean you need to approach them a bit differently. For these people, using techniques that jolt or surprise their thinking pattern – like a sudden mental shock, something confusing, or breaking their usual thought patterns – can be really effective. It's about finding a way to gently bypass that analytical guard so they can explore hypnosis in a way that works for them. We will discuss rapid and instant induction in a later chapter.

Building Trust and Rapport: A key to successfully bypassing the critical factor is building trust and rapport with the client. When a client feels safe and comfortable, their critical factor is more likely to lower its guard, allowing for much more effective subconscious change.

Developing Techniques to Bypass the Critical Factor:

First, metaphors can your best friend. They sneak in ideas in a way that's not too direct. Think of it like using a story to hint at a deeper message. Imagine someone is struggling with letting go of control in their life. You could use the metaphor of a river. You might say, "Imagine your life as a river, flowing naturally. Sometimes, we try to control the direction of the water with our hands, but the river knows its path. By relaxing your grip, you allow the river to flow freely, finding its own way to calmness and clarity." This metaphor gently encourages the idea of releasing control without directly confronting the person's resistance to the concept. It's a softer, more imaginative way to introduce change.

Then there's relaxation – guiding someone to relax bit by bit until they're in a really receptive state is helpful for breaking down barriers of the conscious mind.

Storytelling takes it up a notch. A skilled hypnotherapist is a master at creating and telling detailed stories. You weave in these engaging tales that resonate with the person's experience, and before they know it, they're deeply involved and less guarded. It's like distracting the guard at the gate. Let's say someone is struggling with confidence. You could tell a story about a small seed. This seed, despite being tiny and unseen under the soil, has everything it needs to grow into a magnificent tree. The story would detail the seed's journey, facing challenges like storms and droughts, yet it keeps growing, finding strength within and from the environment. As the person listens, they relate to the seed, seeing their own potential for growth and resilience. This story acts as a distraction for their skeptical mind, allowing the deeper message about confidence and growth to seep in.

Pattern interruption is another ace in the hole. You do or say something unexpected, and it sort of resets their mental state, giving you a window to bypass their skepticism. It's like hitting the refresh button on a webpage. Imagine a client is stuck in a loop of negative self-talk. The therapist, recognizing this pattern, might suddenly change the subject or ask an unexpected or unrelated question to interrupt the pattern or create some confusion. For example, in the middle of a discussion about self-doubt, the therapist might abruptly ask, "What color is the feeling of confidence?" This unexpected shift can momentarily disrupt the client's usual thought process, creating an opening for new perspectives or insights. It's like momentarily switching tracks in a train of thought, providing a chance to redirect the mind towards more positive or productive pathways.

Guided imagery is also great, especially for those who think visually. You help them paint a mental picture, which can lead to some profound insights and changes. It's all about creating a space where they feel safe and open, without that inner critic always on high alert. The key is to mix and match these techniques to fit the person you're working with, keeping it all smooth and natural.

Many of these techniques can be used either in a trance state or in conversational hypnosis. The key is to use all of the tools that you have available to create the biggest positive shift possible for your client.

So, by now, you've got a pretty solid grasp of what hypnosis is all about. It's not just about putting people in a trance; it's a complex, nuanced practice that requires skill, understanding, and a strong ethical compass. Whether you're a budding hypnotist or simply curious about this fascinating field, understanding these principles is key to appreciating the true power and responsibility of working with the subconscious mind.

Chapter 4:
Preparing for Hypnosis

This chapter is all about the crucial steps before starting a hypnosis session. Imagine you're setting up a stage for a play. Every detail matters – from the lighting to the backdrop. Similarly, when working with a client, the environment you create and the trust you build are key. We'll explore how to make your space conducive to relaxation and focus and delve into techniques for establishing rapport with your client. This isn't just about feeling comfortable; it's about creating a foundation that allows for deep, meaningful hypnotic work. Think of it as laying down the tracks for a smooth journey into your subconscious.

Setting the Scene – Crafting a Conducive Environment

For a hypnosis or hypnotherapy session, the physical space is important. Whether you are working out of an office or your home, the physical space is one of the first impressions for your client. You want to create an area that's comfortable, quiet, and distraction-free. Imagine setting up your room with soft lighting that's easy on the eyes, a chair that doesn't rock or swivel, and in my opinion doesn't have arms (arms can interfere with some induction and depending techniques), and an overall peaceful atmosphere. It's all about making a space that naturally feels relaxing, almost like a little sanctuary where you can unwind and focus inward without any outside noise or bother.

The ambiance of the room is a key factor in enhancing the hypnotic experience, going beyond basic comfort. It's important to pay attention to the finer details like the room's temperature, which should be neither too hot nor too cold, creating a neutral, comfortable environment. Lighting plays a critical role too; soft, dimmed lighting can help induce a state of relaxation and calm. The scent is another subtle yet powerful element. The use of aromatherapy, such as lavender or chamomile, can significantly aid in relaxing the client, making them more open to the hypnotic process. These elements combined create an environment that can help facilitate a deeper, more effective hypnotic state.

Incorporating technology and tools can greatly enhance the hypnotic environment as well. Playing soft, soothing, relaxing music can create an auditory backdrop that promotes relaxation and focus. Additionally, tools like a metronome can be very effective. The rhythmic sound of a metronome can aid in inducing a trance state, helping the mind to focus and tune out distractions. These tools, when used skillfully, can add a deeper layer to the hypnotic experience, making it more immersive and effective.

If you are a certified practitioner, displaying your certification certificates in your hypnosis or therapy practice is important for several reasons. First, It provides clients with visible assurance of your qualifications and professional training. This helps build trust and credibility, showing that you're a trained and accredited professional. Having your certificates on display can also offer clients peace of mind, knowing they are in the hands of someone who has the necessary education and skills to provide effective therapy. It's a way of reinforcing your commitment to professional standards and ongoing education in your field and creates a sense of prestige.

The way you dress as a therapist or hypnotist is also quite important. While most people won't expect you to be in a 3-piece suit or formal dress, It's about looking professional, and also about creating a comfortable and reassuring atmosphere for your clients. Your attire should communicate professionalism, respect for the client, and a sense of calm. It's part of the non-verbal communication that helps establish trust and a therapeutic relationship. Dressing appropriately also reflects your own self-respect and dedication to your profession. Think of it as part of the overall therapeutic environment you're creating for your clients.

Building Rapport – The Foundation of Trust

NLP techniques can be one of the most effective and powerful ways to build rapport. You should focus significantly on mirroring, which is a method of subtly matching aspects of another person's behavior. This includes their body language, gestures, posture, and facial expressions. Mirroring isn't about direct imitation but rather *subtly* reflecting these elements. For example, if someone leans forward when speaking, you might do the same. If they cross their legs, you might cross your arms. The goal is to mirror but not make it obvious. Should they suspect that you are imitating them it will destroy rapport. The goal is to create an unconscious sense of familiarity and comfort.

Additionally, mirroring extends to vocal qualities such as tone, volume, and speed of speech. If someone speaks softly and slowly, adjusting your voice to a similar level can create a more harmonious interaction.

Mirroring should be done discreetly and respectfully, ensuring it feels natural and not like mimicry. When executed skillfully, it can significantly enhance the sense of rapport and connection, making communication much more effective.

Pacing and leading is a technique where you first align with someone's current state (pacing) and then gently guide them toward a different mindset (leading). For example, if a client is anxious and speaking quickly, the therapist might start by matching their quick speech and expressing understanding of their anxiety (pacing). Once rapport is established, the therapist gradually adopts a calmer tone and slower speech, encouraging the client to also relax and slow down (leading). This transition helps move the client to a more relaxed state of mind.

Active listening is essential. This means not just hearing the words, but also understanding the emotions and intentions behind them, and reflecting this understanding back to the person.

Using sensory language that aligns with a person's dominant representational system can enhance communication. For instance, if a client frequently uses visual language, like "I see what you mean," or "Let's look at it differently," they likely have a visual dominant system. The therapist can then use visual language in their responses, such as "Picture a place where you feel calm," to better connect with the client's way of processing information.

For someone with an auditory dominant system, using auditory language is effective. If a client often says things like "That sounds right to me" or "I hear what you're saying," they likely process information through hearing. In response, a therapist might use phrases like "Listen to the calmness in your own breath" or "Tell me how that resonates with you."

For a kinesthetic person, who relates more to touch or physical feelings, phrases like "I get a grasp on things" or "That feels right to me" are common. you could respond with language like "Imagine the feeling of tension releasing from your body" or "Focus on the sensation of relaxation spreading through your limbs." These approaches align with the client's natural processing style, creating more effective communication.

Setting Expectations and Easing Anxieties

The hypnotherapy pre-talk is an in-depth conversation that serves as the foundation for a successful session. In this discussion, the therapist will cover several key areas:

Explanation of Hypnosis: The therapist will demystify hypnosis, explaining that it's not like sleep or a loss of consciousness, but a state of focused relaxation. They'll emphasize that the client remains aware and in control.

Addressing Misconceptions: Common myths and Hollywood portrayals of hypnosis might be addressed to ease any fears or misconceptions.

Establishing Goals: The client's objectives for the session are discussed. This helps tailor the hypnotherapy to the client's specific needs.

Discussing the Process: The therapist explains the steps of the session, from induction to the deepening of hypnosis, and the eventual emergence from the hypnotic state.

Consent and Boundaries: Ensuring that the client understands and agrees to the process, and discussing any boundaries or limitations. If any part of your sessions will use ANY physical touch, it is important to get consent.

Personalization: When crafting your script and sessions it's important to ask about the client's preferences for imagery, language, and other aspects of the session to personalize the experience. It is also important to find out about any fears of phobias the client might have. You don't want to be in a position to have them picture them on a beach or lake if they have a fear of drowning!

This conversation sets the stage for a successful and effective hypnotherapy session, ensuring the client is informed, comfortable, and ready to engage with the process.

Mental Preparation – The Hypnotist's Mindset

As a hypnotist, preparing yourself mentally and emotionally before a session is crucial, your job is to be fully present for the client. Prior to each session techniques like mindfulness, meditation, and visualization can help clear your mind ground yourself in the present moment, and stay present and attuned to your client's needs. Meditation can clear your mind, reduce stress, and enhance your focus.

Visualization, imagining the session going well, can boost your confidence and effectiveness. By ensuring you're centered, focused, and fully present, you can create a more effective and empathetic environment for your client. This self-preparation not only benefits your practice but also enhances the overall experience for your clients. You have to fully believe and expect that you will be able to help guide your clients to the change they want. If you don't believe, you won't get the results you want.

Managing expectations is also important for the hypnotist. It's all about being open to different outcomes and flexible in how you approach each session. Sometimes things might not go exactly as planned, and that's okay. It's part of the process. Being adaptable means you can tweak your techniques to better fit the client's needs. It's about going with the flow and making the most of each session, whatever direction it takes.

Preparation is key to the success of a hypnosis session. By creating the right environment and building a strong foundation of trust and rapport, you set the stage for a transformative experience. Remember, the journey of hypnosis is a partnership, and how well you prepare can make all the difference.

Chapter 5:
Suggestibility Tests

Diving into hypnosis without understanding a client's suggestibility is like setting sail without a map. Suggestibility tests are crucial tools in the hypnotist's kit, helping to gauge how a client might respond to hypnosis. This chapter explores why these tests are essential, the different types available, and how to use their results to tailor your hypnosis approach.

Why Suggestibility Tests Matter

Understanding how responsive a client might be to hypnosis is key, and suggestibility tests can help with this. These tests give us a glimpse into how easily a client can slip into a hypnotic state and how they might react to suggestions. It's not about judging their ability, but more about figuring out the best way to approach the hypnotherapy with them. Each client is different, so these tests can guide us in tailoring the session to their unique responsiveness.

Suggestibility tests can be an eye-opener for clients and can be a strong convener. They often help clients see their own potential for entering a hypnotic state, which can be quite empowering. This realization can significantly boost their confidence in the hypnosis process and in their own ability to be hypnotized. It's like giving them a glimpse of their own mental flexibility and receptiveness, which can be both reassuring and motivating as they proceed with the therapy.

Suggestibility tests act like clues, helping to figure out the best way to approach each client's session. Every client's mind is unique, so these tests guide hypnotists in customizing their techniques to fit that individual's specific mental landscape. It's about crafting a hypnotic experience that's just right for them.

Types of Suggestibility Tests

- Verbal Tests: These involve listening and responding to verbal suggestions. We'll explore tests like the 'Lemon' test, where clients respond to suggestions and create physical sensations and responses based on verbal suggestions.
- Non-Verbal Tests: Here, the focus is on response to non-verbal cues. For example, the 'Magnetic fingers' test, where clients are asked to press their hands together and then allow their fingers to be drawn together.

Adapting hypnotic techniques based on a client's level of suggestibility is crucial. For clients who are highly suggestible, direct suggestions might be very effective. They tend to respond well to straightforward, clear instructions. On the other hand, more analytical clients might benefit more from indirect suggestions and storytelling. This approach can bypass their analytical thinking and reach the subconscious more effectively. It's all about matching the technique to the client's way of processing information.

Managing the client's experience during hypnosis involves adjusting your techniques to their needs. For clients who are less suggestible, it might be necessary to spend more time on the induction and deepening phases of the session. This helps them ease into the hypnotic state more gradually and effectively. It's about being patient and using strategies that allow these clients to comfortably transition into a deeper level of relaxation and suggestibility. Tailoring your approach in this way ensures a more positive and effective experience for the client.

A client's beliefs and expectations about hypnosis can shape how they respond to suggestibility tests. This means as a hypnotist, it's important to figure out what's actual suggestibility and what's just their preconceived ideas about being hypnotized. We need to distinguish genuine responsiveness to hypnosis from the influences of these expectations. This understanding helps in crafting a more accurate and effective hypnotherapy approach tailored to the true nature of the client's responsiveness.

Suggestibility tests are a cornerstone in the practice of hypnosis. They're not just a method to gauge a person's responsiveness to hypnotic suggestions, but also a way to build a connection and ease clients into the hypnotic process. Make them fun and don't approach them like it's a true test. You can even call them games for the subconscious. Let's look into four popular suggestibility tests - the Lemon Test, the Book and Balloon Test, the Magnetic Fingers Test, and the Hands Stuck Together Test - detailing each step and offering tips for successful execution.

Suggestibility Test Procedures

1. **The Lemon Test:** Tapping into Imaginative Suggestibility

- Goal: To assess the subject's ability to vividly imagine and physically react to suggestions.
- Procedure:
    - Begin by ensuring the subject is relaxed and seated comfortably. Encourage them to close their eyes.
    - Start painting a detailed picture: they're in a kitchen with a fresh, bright lemon on a cutting board.

- Ask them to visualize slicing the lemon and encourage them to focus on the sensory details: the citrus scent, the feel of the lemon's texture, and the vividness of the color.
  - Instruct them to imagine taking a slice of the lemon and biting into it, emphasizing the sour and tangy taste.
- Tips:
  - Use descriptive language to make the scenario as real as possible.
  - Observe not just facial reactions, but also any subtle body movements.
- Interpreting Responses: Strong physical signs like salivation, puckering, or facial grimacing indicate a high level of imaginative suggestibility.

Here is an effective script for the lemon test:

Introduction:

"Let's try an interesting exercise called the Lemon Suggestibility Test. This will help us explore how your imagination influences your physical responses. Remember, the clearer your imagination, the better. Ready? Let's begin."

Guided Imagery:

"Close your eyes, take a deep, relaxing breath. Picture yourself in your kitchen. Take a moment to notice the details around you – the colors, the layout, perhaps familiar smells. Feel the calmness of being in this familiar space."

Engaging the Senses:

"As you look around your kitchen, you see your refrigerator. Walk over to it and open the door. The light inside gently illuminates the shelves. Your eyes catch a glimpse of a bright yellow lemon. It's sitting there, cool and fresh. Reach out and take the lemon from the fridge. Feel its coolness in your hand, notice its vibrant color and glossy texture."

Interacting with the Lemon:

"Notice the lemon's firmness and the slightly bumpy texture of its skin under your fingers. Now, take a knife and slice the lemon in half. Hear the sound as the knife cuts through the flesh, and watch as the fresh juice starts to glisten in the light."

Tasting the Lemon:

"Pick up one half of the lemon. Observe the juicy interior and the droplets of lemon juice. Bring the lemon half to your mouth and take a big, juicy bite. Feel the burst of tangy juice in your mouth. Taste the sharp, sour flavor on your tongue. Notice how your mouth reacts, perhaps puckering or watering."

Conclusion:

"Place the lemon back down. Take in how you feel in this moment. Breathe deeply again and, when you're ready, gently open your eyes."

Debrief:

"Let's talk about what you just experienced. Did you notice more saliva in your mouth? This exercise demonstrates the power of your imagination and its physical impact. It's a fascinating example of how our minds can influence our bodily reactions."

2. The Book and Balloon Test: Assessing Conflicting Responses

- Goal: To evaluate the subject's responsiveness to suggestions of opposing sensations.
- Procedure:
    - Have the subject stand or sit with arms extended forward, relaxed like a zombie.
    - Suggest a heavy book in one hand (choose a specific book for better visualization) and a light helium balloon tied to the other hand.
    - Gradually intensify the sensations - the book becoming heavier, the balloon pulling the other hand higher.
    - Use vivid descriptions, maybe even mentioning the book's cover texture or the balloon's upward tug.
- Tips:
    - Observe the subject's facial expressions and breathing for signs of engagement.
    - Encourage them to immerse in the experience fully.
- Interpreting Responses: Significant downward movement in one hand and upward in the other suggests a strong physical response to the conflicting suggestions.

The book and balloon sample script

Introduction:

"This is an imaginative exercise known as the Book and Balloon Suggestibility Test. This will help us explore the power of your mind in creating physical sensations and responses. Just relax and let your imagination flow freely. Ready? Let's start."

Setting the Scene:

"First, find a comfortable position and close your eyes. Take a few deep, calming breaths. Allow your body to relax with each exhale. Feel a sense of peace and relaxation washing over you."

Beginning the Imagery:

"Now, imagine that you're standing in a calm, serene place. It can be anywhere you find relaxing. Visualize your surroundings in detail – the colors, the smells, the sounds. Feel the ground under your feet. Extend your arms out, but keep them relaxed, almost like a zombie would stand. Turn your right hand over so the palm is facing up."

Introducing the Objects:

"In your right hand, imagine that you're holding a large, heavy book. It could be an encyclopedia or any large book you can think of. Feel the weight of the book in your hand, its hard cover, and the texture of its pages."

"In your left hand, picture a big bright red, helium-filled balloon tied to your wrist with a light, silky ribbon. The balloon is trying to float up, tugging gently at your wrist. Feel the lightness and the pull of the balloon as it wants to rise into the air. it's almost as if your left arm feels weightless"

Developing the Sensation:

"Notice the book in your right hand starts to feel heavier. It's as if more pages are being added to it. Notice the increasing weight, pulling your arm down, making it harder to keep your hand lifted."

"Now feel the balloon on your left hand is filling with more helium. It's getting larger, lighter, and pulling your left hand up. Feel the contrast between the heavy book and the light, floating balloon."

Enhancing the Experience:

"Imagine the sensations becoming more pronounced. The book is now very heavy, like lead, pulling your right hand down further. The balloon is now so full of helium, effortlessly lifting your left hand higher. Experience this contrast – the heavy weight and the gentle lift."

Conclusion:

"Now, let's gently release the book and the balloon. Feel your arms returning to their normal state, relaxed and comfortable. Take a deep breath in, and as you exhale, allow your imagination to bring you back to the present moment."

Debrief:

"Slowly open your eyes when you're ready. Let's reflect on that experience. How did your arms feel during the exercise? Could you sense the weight of the book and the pull of the balloon? This exercise demonstrates how our mind can create physical sensations purely through imagination."

3. Magnetic Fingers Test: Demonstrating Involuntary Movement

- Goal: To showcase the subject's responsiveness to the idea of involuntary movement.
- Procedure:
  - Ask the subject to extend their arms forward, palms facing each other, fingers slightly apart.
  - Introduce the concept that their fingers are like magnets, inexorably drawing closer.
  - Describe the sensation of the magnetic pull vividly, suggesting it's getting stronger.
  - Watch for the fingers moving together.
- Tips:
  - Focus on gradual and subtle suggestions rather than immediate results.
  - Reinforce the feeling of the pull with each instruction.
- Interpreting Responses: Quick and steady movement of the fingers towards each other is indicative of a higher level of suggestibility.

Magnetic Fingers Script Example

Introduction:

"Let's try an exercise called the Magnetic Fingers Test. This will be a way to see how suggestion and imagination can work together to create physical responses. Just relax, follow my instructions, and let your imagination flow. Ready? Let's start."

Setting the Stage:

"Take a deep breath in, and as you exhale, let your body relax. Feel the tension leaving your muscles. Allow your mind to be calm and receptive."

Engaging the Imagination:

"Clasp your hands tight together, like you're making a fist, but leave your index fingers pointing up and separated by about an inch. Hold your hands up in front of you so you can easily see your fingers."

Introducing the Concept:

"Now, imagine there are powerful magnets on the tips of your index fingers. These magnets are incredibly strong and are starting to pull your fingers toward each other."

Developing the Sensation:

"Focus on your index fingers. Visualize the magnetic force growing more and more potent. Feel the pull, as if these magnets are gently drawing your fingers closer together. It might seem as though your fingers are moving all by themselves, drawn together by this unseen force."

Enhancing the Experience:

"Notice the magnetic pull getting stronger. Your fingers are moving closer, irresistibly attracted to each other. The closer they get, the stronger the pull. Watch as they inch closer and closer, almost as though they're being guided by an invisible force."

Observing the Response:

"Be aware of any sensations in your fingers. You may feel a tingling or warmth as they draw nearer. Let this happen naturally, without forcing it. Just let the imagined magnets do their work."

Conclusion:

"When your fingers finally touch, gently relax your hands. Take a deep breath, and as you breathe out, let go of the image of the magnets. When you feel ready, open your eyes and bring your attention back to the room."

Debrief:

"Let's reflect on that experience. Did you feel the pull of the magnets? How was it to watch your fingers move closer together? This exercise demonstrates how powerful suggestion and imagination can be in influencing our physical movements."

4. Hands Stuck Together Test: Evaluating Response to Direct Physical Suggestion

- Goal: To assess the subject's reaction to direct and physical suggestions.
- Procedure:
    - Instruct the subject to press their palms and fingers together, as if praying.
    - Suggest that their hands are bonding together, becoming one, with the bond strengthening by the second.
    - Enhance the suggestion by describing a feeling of tightness or stickiness between the hands.
    - After a moment, invite them to try and separate their hands.
- Tips:
    - Pay attention to the subject's hand muscle tension and any struggle to separate.
    - Keep your tone confident and assuring throughout the process.

- Interpreting Responses: Difficulty in separating hands, or a significant delay, indicates a strong response to direct physical suggestion.

Hands Stuck Together Sample Script

Introduction:

"Let's do an exercise called the Hands Stuck Together Test. This will allow us to see the power of your mind and its ability to influence your physical experiences through suggestion. All you need to do is follow my instructions and allow your imagination to fully engage in the process."

Setting the Stage:

"Sit comfortably and relax. Close your eyes and take a few deep breaths. With each exhale, feel yourself becoming more and more relaxed. Let your mind be open and receptive to this experience."

Engaging the Imagination:

"Now, with your eyes closed, bring your hands together in front of you. Clasp them tightly, interlocking your fingers. Press your palms together firmly. Your hands are becoming one unit, tightly bound together."

Introducing the Concept:

"Imagine now that a strong glue is being applied to your clasped hands. This is a special kind of glue, incredibly strong and fast-acting. Feel the glue binding your hands together, sealing them tight."

Developing the Sensation:

"As you focus on your hands, this glue is becoming stronger, making it harder and harder to separate your fingers and palms. Your hands feel like they are securely stuck together as if they are carved from one solid piece of wood. Try to feel the texture and strength of this glue, reinforcing the bond between your hands."

Enhancing the Experience:

"Your hands are now completely stuck. The more you try to pull them apart, the more you find them firmly glued together. The harder you try, the more they become stuck. It's as though they are locked in place. The glue is unyielding, holding your hands tightly."

Testing the Suggestion:

"Take a moment to test the strength of this bond. Gently try to pull your hands apart and notice the resistance. Feel the strength of the glue keeping your hands firmly together. Observe the effort it takes to even attempt to separate them."

Conclusion:

"Now, imagine a warm, soothing liquid being poured over your hands, dissolving the glue. Slowly, the bond begins to weaken. Your hands start to feel looser. Gradually, you can start moving your fingers again. The glue is completely dissolved, and you can easily and gently separate your hands."

"Take a deep breath in, and as you exhale, allow your hands to relax and separate. When you're ready, open your eyes, returning your focus to the room."

Debrief:

"Let's discuss what you experienced. Were your hands feeling stuck together? How did it feel trying to separate them? This exercise demonstrates the incredible power of suggestion and the mind's ability to create physical sensations and responses."

Mastering suggestibility tests is crucial for every hypnotist, the success of your hypnosis sessions depends on getting the feedback you need during these tests. They not only gauge responsiveness but also help in creating a bond of trust and expectation between the hypnotist and the subject. Remember, the goal is not to challenge the subject but to guide them into a deeper understanding of their own mind's potential. Practice these tests with sensitivity and care, and you'll find them invaluable in your hypnotherapy practice.

Chapter 6:
Induction Techniques

The hypnosis induction is the first step in guiding someone into a hypnotic state. In this chapter, we will look deep into various induction techniques. This includes detailed instructions and tips to make sure you're practicing these methods effectively. Whether you're just starting out or you're already experienced in hypnotherapy, understanding the subtle details of different induction techniques is essential. It's these nuances that can make or break the success of a hypnosis session, leading to truly transformative experiences for your clients.

Progressive Relaxation Induction

Progressive Relaxation Induction is a popular technique in hypnosis that involves guiding the person into a state of deep relaxation, step by step. This method focuses on relaxing each muscle group in the body gradually, often starting from the toes and moving upwards. As the physical body relaxes, the mind follows, allowing the individual to reach a deeper state of hypnotic relaxation. The therapist's calm and steady voice, along with guided imagery and suggestions, helps facilitate this process. It's particularly effective for people new to hypnosis or those who find it hard to relax. Most new or inexperienced hypnotherapists will have the most success with progressive relaxation techniques.

- Procedure:

    Create a Relaxing Atmosphere: Ensure the room is quiet and comfortable. Soft lighting and a comfortable chair (that doesn't rock or swivel) can enhance the relaxation experience.

Encourage the subject to take deep, slow breaths. Guide them to focus on the rhythm of their breathing, perhaps synchronizing breaths with a calm, rhythmic verbal cue.

Starting at the toes, instruct the subject to tense each muscle group for a few seconds and then release. Gradually move up through the body - feet, ankles, calves, and so on, up to the facial muscles.

Deepening Relaxation: With each muscle group relaxed, reinforce the sense of deepening calm. You might say, "As your muscles relax, your mind relaxes even more deeply."

- Tips: Be patient and move at a pace that matches the subject's response. The goal is a gradual deepening of relaxation.

Visualization Induction

A visualization Induction is a technique where the client is guided to imagine a peaceful and calming scene or scenario. This process helps the client to relax deeply and enter a hypnotic state. The hypnotist typically describes a serene environment in detail, encouraging the client to engage their senses in the imagined scene. This could involve picturing a tranquil beach, a quiet forest, or any other setting that evokes relaxation. As the client becomes more absorbed in the visualization, they become more receptive to suggestions, making this a highly effective method for inducing hypnosis.

- Procedure:

Setting the Scene: Start by guiding the subject to envision a place where they feel peaceful and happy. This could be a beach, a forest, a garden, or any place they find relaxing. (you should already have this information based on your previous conversation with the client)

Engaging the Senses: Encourage them to explore this place with all their senses. Ask them to notice the sounds, the scents, the sights, and the textures around them.

Deepening the Experience: Introduce elements that symbolize relaxation, such as a gentle breeze, the warmth of the sun, or the sensation of water.

Transition to Hypnosis: As they become more absorbed, suggest that with each breath and step in this place, they are moving deeper into a state of hypnosis.

- Tips: Use rich, descriptive language. The more vivid the scene, the more effective the induction.

Rapid Induction Techniques

If you have ever seen a stage or street hypnotist, you've likely seen them use a rapid or instant induction technique.

The benefits of these techniques are often overlooked or not used in a clinical setting, but the reality is that they can be extremely effective in clinical hypnotherapy.

In clinical hypnosis, the efficiency of rapid inductions is a key advantage. With therapy sessions often constrained by time, these quick methods allow for more of the session to be devoted to therapeutic interventions, addressing the client's specific needs. They are particularly useful for reducing initial client anxiety, swiftly bypassing the critical conscious mind to facilitate a more receptive state for the session. This heightened focus can potentially make the therapy more effective. Rapid inductions also allow the hypnotherapist to immediately gauge a client's responsiveness, enabling real-time adjustments to the session approach. Demonstrating the ability to induce hypnosis rapidly can also build trust and rapport, enhancing the client's confidence in the hypnotist's skills.

These techniques quickly induce a hypnotic state, often in a matter of seconds or minutes. These techniques are typically more direct and assertive, utilizing elements of surprise or confusion to bypass the analytical mind. They might involve sudden, unexpected commands or actions that focus and narrow the client's attention rapidly. These methods require skill and experience to execute effectively and are best used by experienced hypnotherapists.

Often when working with a client I will use one of the other techniques on the first session unless they have demonstrated that they are highly suggestable. Rapid inductions can have great results, but strong rapport is critical.

- Procedure:
  Preparation: Build rapport quickly and ensure the subject is comfortable with a rapid approach. Explain that the process will be quick but relaxing.

  Startle Technique: Use a safe, unexpected gesture, like a gentle tap on the shoulder or a sudden clap, followed immediately by a direct command like "Sleep!"

Immediate Deepening: Follow up with rapid deepening techniques, such as counting down from 10 to 1, each number leading them deeper into hypnosis.

Reinforcement: Quickly reinforce the state with suggestions of relaxation and calmness.

- Tips: Be confident and assertive. The sudden contrast between the startle and the calming follow-up is key to this method's success. After giving the "Sleep" command it is critical to keep talking in a calm voice. I usually use the suggestions of "Drifting, dreaming, dropping, falling, the more you relax the better you feel and the better you feel the deeper you relax" Then go into a deepener.

The Elman Induction

The Elman Induction is a well-known hypnotherapy technique developed by Dave Elman. It's known for quickly inducing a deep state of hypnosis. While not as quick as a rapid induction, it typically only takes 3-5 minutes to get the client in a deep trance. The process typically involves guiding the client through several stages of relaxation, often starting with the eyes and moving through the body. It includes specific suggestions for deepening relaxation and testing the depth of hypnosis. The Elman Induction is particularly appreciated for its structure and effectiveness, making it a popular choice among many hypnotists. The Elman induction is also very effective when working remotely over Zoom or other video conferencing. You would simply remove the physical touch element.

- Procedure:

   Instruct the subject to close their eyes and focus on letting go of tension. Have them imagine relaxing them to the point that the eyes just won't open. When they are confident that they have relaxed them to a point where they won't open, have them test them. After 2-3 seconds tell them to stop testing and their eyes return to a relaxed state.

   Have the client imagine that relaxation spreading throughout the body.

   Tell the client that you are going to lift their arm and that arm will be "As limp as a wet dish rag". Tell them when you drop their arm in the lap they will go deeper into relaxation. Do this twice, or once with each arm.

   Instruct the client to open their eyes momentarily and instruct them that when they close them again they will go 10 times deeper into relaxation. When they open their eyes have your hand in front of their face so that the eyes can't focus. I normally do this 2-3 times.

   Tell them that now that they've relaxed the body, we are going to relax the mind. Tell them that you are going to have them count backward from 100. When they start counting tell them with each number to double the relaxation, letting your mind and body become twice as relaxed as the moment before.

Perhaps when you reach 98 or 97 you might find that the numbers start to fade away, becoming more and more difficult to remember or vanish altogether.

allow each number to drift out of your mind. They become less and less important. The only thing that matters is this deep sense of relaxation.

If you reach a point where the next number seems to vanish, just let it go. It's a wonderful sign that you are deeply relaxed and focused.

Now deepen the trance.
Guide them to imagine a relaxing scenario, like descending a staircase, with each step taking them deeper into relaxation.

- Tips: The pace is important here. Keep your instructions clear and steady, and observe the subject's responses to adjust your pace accordingly.

Each induction technique offers a unique pathway to the hypnotic state. Understanding and mastering the details of these procedures allows for flexibility and adaptability in your practice. Remember, the goal is not just to induce hypnosis but to create a comfortable and trusting environment in which the subject feels safe and open to the experience. Practice, patience, and a responsive approach are key to mastering these techniques.

Chapter 7:
Deepening Techniques

Once a subject is induced into a hypnotic state, the next step is deepening the trance to achieve a more profound and effective level of hypnosis. This chapter explores various strategies to deepen the hypnotic trance, along with recognizing and working with different levels of trance. We'll provide specific examples to illustrate these techniques in action.

The Art of Deepening Trance

- The Staircase Method: This classic technique involves guiding the subject to imagine descending a staircase, with each step taking them deeper into relaxation. You can enhance this imagery by describing a sense of increasing heaviness with each step or the feeling of sinking deeper into calmness.
- Counting Down: Counting down from 10 or 20 is a straightforward method. With each number, suggest that the subject is becoming more relaxed and more deeply hypnotized. For instance, "With each number I count, feel yourself drifting deeper into a state of complete relaxation."
- Use of Imagery: Create a serene scene, like a garden or a peaceful beach. Describe the scene in rich detail, focusing on sensory experiences. For example, "Imagine the soft, warm sand under your feet, taking you deeper into tranquility with every step."

Recognizing Levels of Trance

- Light Trance: Indicated by physical relaxation and a calm demeanor. The subject might still be very aware of their surroundings.

- Medium Trance: Characterized by more profound relaxation, slower breathing, and less awareness of the physical environment.
- Deep Trance: The subject is highly responsive to suggestions, deeply relaxed, and may have reduced conscious awareness of their surroundings.

Tailoring Techniques to Trance Levels

- For Light Trance: Focus on simple, soothing suggestions and gentle imagery to encourage deeper relaxation.
- For Medium Trance: Utilize more direct suggestions and potentially introduce therapeutic concepts or imagery.
- For Deep Trance: This level is suitable for more complex suggestions and therapeutic interventions.

Specific Examples of Deepening Techniques:

Ocean Waves Visualization: "Imagine each wave of the ocean bringing you deeper into relaxation, each wave gently carrying you further into a calm and peaceful state."

Color Visualization: "Visualize a color that represents relaxation to you. With each breath, imagine this color washing over you, taking you deeper into a state of hypnotic trance."

Elevator Technique: "Imagine you're in an elevator, smoothly descending. With each level down, you feel more relaxed, more at ease, and more deeply hypnotized."

Relaxing Body Scan: Guide the subject through a body scan, suggesting that each part of their body is becoming heavier and more relaxed, deepening their trance with each moment.

Use of Metaphors: Employ metaphors like a river flowing smoothly into the sea, symbolizing the transition from a lighter to a deeper state of trance.

Reinforcing Depth

- Affirmation of Depth: Affirm the depth of trance by suggesting that the subject is now in a very deep and comfortable state of hypnosis.
- Feedback Loop: Encourage the subject to signal their level of trance, either verbally or with a finger lift, and use this feedback to adjust your deepening techniques.

Mastering deepening techniques is crucial for effective hypnotherapy. By recognizing the different levels of trance and tailoring your approach, you can facilitate a more meaningful and therapeutic hypnotic experience. Practice, observation, and sensitivity to the subject's responses are key to enhancing your skill in deepening trance states.

Chapter 8:

Suggestion and Communication - Enhancing Hypnotic Effectiveness

In hypnosis, the power of suggestion coupled with effective communication forms the backbone of a successful session. This chapter offers a deeper exploration into the art of crafting suggestions and the nuances of both verbal and non-verbal communication, crucial for establishing a transformative hypnotic experience. We will also delve into the use of metaphors and provide detailed examples to illustrate these concepts.

The Art of Crafting Effective Suggestions

- Elements of a Good Suggestion:
    - Specificity: Tailor suggestions to address specific issues or goals of the subject. For instance, for someone seeking to quit smoking, a suggestion could be, "You will find yourself craving fresh air more than a cigarette."
    - Immediacy: Use the present tense to make suggestions immediate and relevant. For example, "You are becoming more confident with each passing moment."
    - Positive Outcomes: Focus on positive changes and outcomes. Instead of focusing on what the subject should avoid, concentrate on what they should feel or do.
    - Sensory Detail: Engage the senses in your suggestions. For instance, "Feel the warmth of confidence spreading through your body."

Creating Compound Suggestions: These are suggestions that link several positive outcomes or steps. For example, "As you breathe deeply and relax, you feel a sense of confidence building inside you, preparing you to face any challenge with calmness and clarity."

Mastering Verbal Communication

- Voice Modulation: The hypnotist's voice should be soothing yet firm, providing comfort while guiding the trance. Practice varying your tone, pitch, and volume to convey different emotions and deepen the trance.
- The Language of Hypnosis: Use language that is vivid, imaginative, and rich in sensory detail. Utilize metaphors, analogies, and stories to create a more engaging and relatable hypnotic experience.
- Directive vs. Permissive Language: Some subjects respond better to direct commands ("You are feeling relaxed"), while others may prefer permissive language ("Perhaps you can feel yourself becoming more and more relaxed"). Being able to switch between these styles based on the subject's response is crucial.

Examples of Metaphors in Script Crafting:

The Safe Haven Metaphor: "Imagine yourself in a safe haven, a place where nothing can disturb you. This haven is your mind's creation, perfect for your relaxation and healing."

The Mountain Metaphor: "See yourself climbing a mountain. With each step, you leave behind anxieties, moving higher towards the peak of clarity and calmness."

The Garden Metaphor: "Envision a beautiful garden, your inner place of peace. Each flower represents a quality you wish to nurture - confidence, calmness, joy."

The Flowing River Metaphor: "Imagine your thoughts are like a river, flowing smoothly and effortlessly. Obstacles in the river represent your stresses and worries, and as the river flows, it effortlessly washes these obstacles away, leaving your mind clear and serene."

The Protective Shield Metaphor: "Envision a shield surrounding you, glowing with a calming light. This shield protects you from negativity and stress. Each breath strengthens this shield, letting only positivity and peace filter through."

The Blossoming Flower Metaphor: "Picture a bud in a garden, representing your inner potential. With each suggestion, feel the bud blossoming, revealing a beautiful flower. This flower symbolizes your growth, opening up to new possibilities and confidence."

The Calm Lake Metaphor: "Visualize a tranquil lake, its surface smooth and undisturbed. This lake mirrors your mind, becoming more peaceful and calm. Each gentle wave soothes your thoughts, bringing deeper levels of relaxation and clarity."

The Sunrise Metaphor: "Imagine the first light of sunrise, signaling the start of a new day. With each ray of light, feel a sense of renewal and hope. This sunrise brings with it a day filled with potential and positive energy."

The Journey Metaphor: "See yourself on a path, stretching out before you. Each step on this path is a step forward in your life. Feel the excitement of journeying towards your goals, leaving behind any barriers or limitations."

The Balancing Scales Metaphor: "Picture a set of scales, representing the balance in your life. Each suggestion helps to tip the scales towards harmony and equilibrium, balancing your emotions and bringing a sense of inner stability."

The Ancient Tree Metaphor: "Envision an ancient, sturdy tree. You are like this tree, grounded and strong. Your roots extend deep into the ground, giving you stability. With each breath, feel more connected to your sources of strength and resilience."

The Cozy Cabin Metaphor: "Imagine a cozy cabin in the woods, a safe and warm place. This cabin is your mind's sanctuary, where you can relax fully and recharge. In this cabin, you find peace and comfort, away from the outside world."

The Light Feather Metaphor: "Visualize a light feather floating gently in the breeze. This feather represents your worries and concerns, which are now being carried away by the wind, leaving you light, carefree, and relaxed."

Techniques to Reinforce Suggestions

- Layered Suggestions: Embed suggestions within a story or metaphor. This can make the suggestion more palatable and less direct.

Example: The Journey to Inner Strength

> *Imagine yourself on a journey through a dense forest. This forest represents your life, filled with both challenges and opportunities. As you walk along the winding path, you notice the trees around you, some tall and strong, others leaning or swaying. These trees symbolize the various aspects of your thoughts and emotions.*
>
> *You come across a tree that stands tall and unwavering, its branches reaching confidently towards the sky. This tree represents your inner strength and resilience. With each step closer to it, you begin to feel a sense of determination and self-assuredness growing within you.*
>
> *As you stand beside this mighty tree, you realize that you, too, possess the same unwavering strength deep within yourself. It's always been there, waiting for you to tap into it. With this newfound understanding, you continue your journey through the forest, feeling more self-assured and confident with each step.*

In this metaphor, the suggestion of inner strength is embedded within the story of the forest journey. By comparing the subject's inner strength to the sturdy tree, the suggestion becomes more palatable and indirect. The subject is encouraged to connect with their inner strength in a symbolic and meaningful way, making it a powerful and enduring suggestion.

- Future Pacing is a detailed process where you guide a client to vividly imagine experiencing the positive outcomes of therapy in their future life. For instance, if a client seeks confidence in public speaking, you would lead them to visualize a future scenario where they are speaking confidently and effortlessly in front of an audience. They would imagine the details – the setting, the audience's positive reactions, the feeling of confidence in their voice, and the sense of accomplishment afterward. This visualization makes the desired change feel tangible and achievable, reinforcing the therapy's suggestions. By mentally 'experiencing' these positive outcomes, the client's subconscious is more inclined to believe in and work towards these changes in their real life.

- Anchoring in hypnotherapy involves creating a link between a physical gesture or word and a specific emotional state. For instance, you might guide a client to touch their thumb and forefinger together while they are feeling particularly relaxed and calm during a session. This gesture becomes an 'anchor' for that feeling of calmness. Later, when they need to evoke this sense of calm, repeating the gesture can help bring back the associated feelings of relaxation. This technique is a powerful tool for helping clients access desired states or responses on demand.

- Symbolic Imagery: Utilize imagery that symbolizes personal growth or overcoming challenges. For example, "Imagine climbing a hill. With each step, you feel lighter, leaving behind any burdens. Reaching the top symbolizes achieving your goal, feeling a sense of accomplishment and freedom."

- Positive Association: Link positive feelings or states to everyday actions. For instance, "Each morning when you see the sun, you will feel a renewed sense of energy and optimism."

- Sensory Engagement: Engage multiple senses in suggestions. For example, "Imagine the scent of a pine forest, the sound of rustling leaves, and the feeling of the cool, refreshing air. These sensations fill you with peace and tranquility."

- Echo Technique: Repeat key phrases or suggestions. This repetition helps cement the ideas. For instance, "You are calm and in control... calm and in control... calm and in control..."

- Reframing: Alter the subject's perspective on a problem. For example, "What once felt like a challenge, now appears as an opportunity for growth and learning."

- Guided Storytelling: Create a story where the protagonist (representing the subject) overcomes obstacles or achieves desired changes. This can help the subject visualize their success.

- Progressive Success: Suggest a gradual improvement in the subject's condition. For example, "Each day, you find yourself managing stress more effectively than the day before."

- Contrast Technique: Contrast the undesirable state with the desired state. For example, "Where once there was stress, now there is calm. Where there was doubt, now there's confidence."

- Affirmation of Ability: Repeatedly affirm the subject's ability to achieve their goal. For instance, "You have the strength and the willpower to make positive changes in your life."

- Personal Empowerment: Emphasize the subject's control over their change. For example, "You hold the power to transform your thoughts and actions in a way that benefits you."

- Metaphorical Journey: Take the subject on a metaphorical journey that parallels their real-life journey. For instance, "Imagine walking down a path that represents your life. Notice how the path becomes smoother as you progress, just like your journey towards your goal."

- Conditional Suggestions: These are suggestions that become effective under certain conditions. For example, "Whenever you feel the urge to smoke, you will instead feel a strong motivation to drink water or take a deep breath."

- Visualization of the Future Self: Guide the subject to visualize their future self, in a dissociated state, having achieved their goals. This helps to create a strong mental image of success.

Effective suggestion and communication in hypnosis require practice, empathy, and a deep understanding of the subject's needs and responses. By mastering the art of suggestion, enhancing your verbal and non-verbal communication skills, and effectively utilizing metaphors, you can significantly improve the results of your sessions. Remember, each subject is unique, and flexibility in your approach is key to a successful hypnotic experience.

Chapter 9:
Transforming Lives

Let's jump in and bring this all together so that we can start making some transformations. This is all about making big, meaningful changes - whether in your life or in the lives of your clients. We're about to explore some really powerful techniques and strategies that can seriously shake things up for the better. But this isn't just about tweaking a few things here and there. We're talking about deep, life-changing shifts that open new doors, help us understand ourselves better, and unlock potential that might have seemed out of reach before. So, get ready for an exciting ride. Every step we take is a move towards a more fulfilling life, whether that's for you or for the people you're helping as clients.

Once you've figured out what issue or change you're going to work on, it's time to think about what kind of suggestions will really hit home. Think about what makes this situation unique and how you can craft your approach to make a real impact.

The order of the hypnosis session should be:

1. Pre-talk
2. Induction
3. Deepener
4. Therapy (your script)
5. Future Pace
6. Re-orientation
7. Post session talk

The following scripts and suggestions will help you formulate suggestions to give after deepening.

Techniques for Using Hypnotherapy for Stress Reduction

Hypnotherapy is a powerful tool for managing and reducing stress. By guiding clients (or yourself) into a deep state of relaxation and accessing the subconscious mind, hypnotherapy can help alleviate stress, promote relaxation, and build resilience. Here are some techniques commonly used in hypnotherapy for stress reduction:

1. Progressive Muscle Relaxation (PMR): This technique involves guiding the individual to progressively tense and then release different muscle groups in the body. It promotes physical relaxation and reduces tension.

- *Script Example:* "As you breathe in, gently tense the muscles in your arms, feeling the tension. Now, as you exhale, release that tension, allowing your muscles to become loose and relaxed."

2. Visualization: Visualization techniques encourage individuals to create mental images of peaceful and calming scenes. This can transport them away from stress-inducing thoughts and emotions.

- *Script Example:* "Imagine yourself in a serene garden. Picture the vibrant colors, feel the warmth of the sun on your skin, and hear the gentle rustling of leaves. As you immerse yourself in this tranquil place, your stress melts away."

3. Breathing Techniques: Hypnotherapy can teach deep breathing exercises to calm the nervous system and reduce stress.

- *Script Example:* "Take a slow, deep breath in through your nose, allowing your lungs to fill with calming fresh air. Hold it for a moment, and then exhale slowly through your mouth releasing any stress or tension on the exhale. With each breath, you become more and more relaxed."

4. Positive Affirmations: Affirmations can reprogram the mind with positive beliefs and counteract negative thought patterns associated with stress.

- *Script Example:* "In your mind, repeat after me: 'I am calm and at peace. I handle stress with grace and resilience. I am in control of my emotions.'"

5. Guided Imagery: This technique involves guiding individuals through a mental journey to a peaceful place where they can visualize themselves free from stress.

- *Script Example:* "Picture yourself on a serene beach. You can feel the soft sand beneath your feet, the gentle breeze on your skin, and the sound of waves calming your mind. In this moment, stress has no place."

6. Self-Hypnosis: Teach individuals how to induce a state of self-hypnosis on their own. They can use self-hypnosis whenever they encounter stress triggers.

- *Script Example:* "You have the power to enter a state of deep relaxation whenever you choose. By counting down from 5 to 1, you can quickly enter a state of calm and tranquility."

7. Stress Reduction Anchoring: Create an anchor, such as touching two fingers together, that individuals can use to trigger a state of relaxation whenever they need it.

- *Script Example:* "As you touch your thumb and forefinger together, you instantly activate a sense of relaxation. You can use this anchor whenever you feel stressed to bring yourself back to a state of calm."

8. Reframing Negative Thoughts: Help individuals reframe negative thoughts and perceptions about stressors, allowing them to see challenges in a more positive light.

- *Script Example:* "Think of stress as a signal from your body, guiding you to take care of yourself. It's an opportunity for growth and self-improvement."

When using these techniques in hypnotherapy for stress reduction, it's essential to tailor the approach to the individual's needs and preferences. Hypnotherapy sessions can be highly personalized to address specific stressors and promote relaxation and emotional well-being. Through consistent practice, individuals can develop resilience to stress and enjoy a more balanced and harmonious life.

Techniques for Using Hypnotherapy for Anxiety and Depression

Hypnotherapy is a valuable approach for addressing anxiety and depression, as it can access the subconscious mind to reframe negative thought patterns, promote relaxation, and instill positive beliefs and coping strategies. Here are techniques commonly used in hypnotherapy for anxiety and depression:

1. Positive Affirmations: Affirmations are powerful tools for shifting negative thought patterns. Hypnopractitioners can guide individuals to repeat positive affirmations that counteract self-doubt and pessimism.

- *Script Example for Anxiety:* "Repeat after me: 'I am calm and confident. I can handle any situation with ease and grace.'"
- *Script Example for Depression:* "Say to yourself: 'I am worthy of happiness and love. Each day, I embrace the joy in my life.'"

2. Cognitive Restructuring: This technique helps individuals identify and challenge irrational or negative beliefs that contribute to anxiety and depression. Hypnotherapy can assist in replacing these beliefs with more constructive ones.

- *Script Example for Anxiety:* "Let's explore the thoughts that make you anxious. Are they based on facts or assumptions? We will reframe these thoughts to reflect reality."
- *Script Example for Depression:* "We'll work on recognizing when your thoughts become negative or self-critical. We'll replace them with positive and self-affirming beliefs."

3. Visualization and Imagery: Guided imagery can transport

individuals to a place of inner calm and positivity.

- *Script Example for Anxiety:* "Imagine a serene lake. See your anxious thoughts as ripples on the surface. As you breathe deeply, the water becomes still, and your mind becomes calm."
- *Script Example for Depression:* "Visualize a beautiful sunrise, representing new beginnings and hope. As the sun rises, you feel a sense of renewal and optimism."

4. Progressive Relaxation: Similar to stress reduction,

progressive muscle relaxation techniques can help release

physical tension associated with anxiety and depression.

- *Script Example for Anxiety:* "Tighten and then release your muscles, starting from your toes and working up to your head. With each release, let go of anxious feelings."
- *Script Example for Depression:* "As you relax your body, envision releasing emotional weight and burdens. With each breath, you become lighter and more free."

5. Inner Child Healing: For individuals with unresolved past traumas contributing to anxiety or depression, hypnotherapy can facilitate inner child healing.

- *Script Example for Anxiety:* "Imagine yourself as a child. Embrace that inner child, offering love and reassurance. Healing the past will ease your anxiety."
- *Script Example for Depression:* "Connect with your inner child, offering comfort and support. Healing these wounds will bring greater emotional well-being."

6. Future Progression: Help individuals visualize a positive future, free from anxiety or depression, to create motivation and a sense of hope.

- *Script Example for Anxiety:* "Imagine yourself confidently handling challenging situations. Picture a future where anxiety no longer controls your life."
- *Script Example for Depression:* "Visualize a future where you wake up each day with a sense of purpose and joy. This is the future we're working towards."

7. Anchoring Techniques: Create anchors (physical or mental cues) that individuals can use to instantly access a state of calm and positivity when needed.

- *Script Example for Anxiety:* "Touch your thumb and forefinger together while experiencing a calm state. This anchor will help you manage anxiety in the moment."

- *Script Example for Depression:* "By visualizing a specific symbol in your mind, you can instantly lift your mood and access a happier state."

These techniques can be adapted and combined in personalized hypnotherapy sessions to address the unique needs and challenges of individuals dealing with anxiety and depression. By working with a skilled hypnopractitioner, individuals can experience profound shifts in their thought patterns, emotions, and overall well-being, leading to a more positive and fulfilling life.

Techniques for Using Hypnotherapy to Overcome Fears and Phobias

Hypnotherapy offers effective methods for conquering fears and phobias by accessing the subconscious mind and reshaping negative associations. It enables individuals to confront their fears in a secure and controlled environment. Here are techniques, including the double dissociation method, commonly employed in hypnotherapy for overcoming fears and phobias:

1. Systematic Desensitization: This gradual exposure technique starts with the least anxiety-inducing scenario and progresses to more challenging ones. In hypnotherapy, it can be enhanced by incorporating relaxation and dissociation techniques.

- *Script Example with Dissociation:* "As you enter a state of deep relaxation, imagine yourself observing a movie screen in front of you. On the screen, you see a distant image of the feared object or situation. Notice how detached and calm you feel as you watch the scene unfold."

2. Hypnotic Imagery and Visualization: Hypnopractitioners guide individuals to create positive mental images and associations with the feared object or situation.

- *Script Example with Dissociation:* "Imagine stepping into a movie theater where you watch yourself confidently facing the feared situation on the big screen. Observe how you, as the viewer, remain relaxed and unaffected by the scenario."

3. Regression Therapy: Regression techniques can uncover past experiences or traumas underlying the fear. Using double dissociation, individuals can view these memories from an observer's perspective to reduce emotional intensity.

- *Script Example with Dissociation:* "Imagine floating above your younger self in that past moment when the fear first took root. You are an observer, detached from the emotions of the past. We will work on healing and reframing this memory."

4. Positive Affirmations: Positive affirmations are employed to reprogram the subconscious mind, replacing fear-based beliefs with empowering ones.

- *Script Example with Dissociation:* "In your mind's eye, picture yourself in front of a mirror. As you say the affirmations, notice how the 'you' in the mirror smiles with confidence, reinforcing these positive beliefs."

5. Anchoring Techniques: Create anchors (physical or mental cues) that individuals associate with a sense of calm and confidence, which they can use when facing the feared object or situation.

- *Script Example:* "As you touch your thumb and forefinger together, imagine watching this action from a distance. Observe how it connects you to a feeling of strength and courage."

6. Exposure Therapy: Simulate exposure to the feared object or situation through hypnosis, allowing the individual to practice managing their fear response.

- *Script Example with Dissociation:* "In your mind, imagine being inside a protective bubble. Outside the bubble is the feared object or situation. As you watch it from this safe perspective, notice how your anxiety lessens."

7. Reframing Negative Associations: Help individuals reinterpret their fears by changing the way they perceive and think about the feared object or situation.

- *Script Example with Dissociation:* "Imagine seeing the feared object or situation through a pair of glasses. These glasses transform it into something harmless and non-threatening, altering your perception."

8. Future Pacing: Guide individuals to visualize themselves confidently facing the feared situation in the future, reinforcing positive changes.

- *Script Example with Dissociation:* "Imagine standing on a stage, addressing an audience without fear. Watch yourself from a balcony seat in the theater, observing your poised and confident self."

These techniques, enhanced by double dissociation, create a sense of detachment and perspective, allowing individuals to observe their fears from a safe and empowered vantage point. By consistently applying these methods in hypnotherapy sessions, individuals can gradually overcome their fears and phobias, regaining control over their emotions and experiences.

Techniques in Hypnosis for Weight Loss

Hypnosis can be a powerful tool for supporting weight loss efforts by addressing both the psychological and behavioral aspects of overeating and unhealthy eating habits. Here are some effective techniques used in hypnotherapy for weight loss

1. Cognitive Restructuring: Hypnopractitioners help individuals identify and reframe negative thought patterns related to food, body image, and self-worth. By replacing self-criticism with self-acceptance and positive affirmations, clients can develop a healthier relationship with food.

- *Example Script:* "Replace thoughts of 'I can't resist that dessert' with 'I have the power to make healthy choices.' You are in control of your eating habits."

2. Visualization and Imagery: Guided imagery can assist clients in creating mental images of their ideal body and health. By visualizing themselves as fit, healthy, and confident, individuals can motivate themselves to make better food choices.

- *Example Script:* "Picture yourself standing in front of a mirror, seeing a slimmer, healthier version of yourself. Feel the joy and confidence that comes with this transformation."

3. Mindful Eating: Hypnotherapy can encourage mindful eating practices, which involve paying close attention to the sensory experience of eating, such as taste, texture, and satisfaction. This helps clients eat more slowly and recognize when they're full.

- *Example Script:* "As you take each bite, savor the flavors and textures. Listen to your body's signals of hunger and fullness. Eating mindfully allows you to enjoy food without overeating."

4. Behavior Modification: Hypnopractitioners work with clients to identify specific behaviors that contribute to overeating, such as emotional eating or mindless snacking. Techniques like anchoring can be used to create cues for healthier habits.

- *Example Script:* "When you feel stressed, instead of reaching for unhealthy snacks, use your anchor to remind yourself to take a deep breath and choose a healthier option."

5. Stress Reduction: Stress is a common trigger for overeating. Hypnotherapy helps individuals manage stress through relaxation techniques, reducing the need to turn to food for comfort.

- *Example Script:* "Imagine a place of perfect calm and relaxation. Whenever stress arises, you can mentally transport yourself to this peaceful oasis."

6. Portion Control: Hypnotherapy can assist clients in developing a sense of portion control. By visualizing appropriate serving sizes and feeling satisfied with smaller portions, individuals can reduce calorie intake.

- *Example Script:* "Imagine your plate with the perfect portion sizes. As you eat, you feel comfortably full with these portions, and you don't need to eat more."

7. Self-Esteem and Body Image: Improving self-esteem and body image is essential for weight loss success. Hypnotherapy can help individuals feel more confident and positive about themselves.

- *Example Script:* "You are worthy of love and acceptance just as you are. Embrace your body with love and gratitude as you work towards your health goals."

8. Goal Setting: Setting clear and achievable weight loss goals is crucial. Hypnotherapy can assist in creating a mental roadmap for success and maintaining motivation.

- *Example Script:* "See yourself reaching your weight loss goals step by step. Each small achievement brings you closer to your ultimate success."

9. Building Healthy Habits: Hypnotherapy reinforces the formation of healthy eating and exercise habits by embedding positive suggestions into the subconscious mind.

- *Example Script:* "Your desire for healthy foods and regular exercise grows stronger every day. You naturally choose foods that nourish your body, and exercise becomes a joyful habit."

10. Future Pacing: Visualizing a future where weight loss goals have been achieved can provide motivation and reinforce commitment to healthier choices.

- *Example Script:* "Imagine yourself a year from now, living your ideal healthy life. Feel the pride and happiness of your success."

These techniques, when integrated into a comprehensive hypnotherapy program, can support individuals in their weight loss journey by addressing the underlying psychological factors that contribute to overeating and promoting healthier behaviors and attitudes towards food and body image. It's important to work with a skilled hypnopractitioner who can tailor the approach to the individual's specific needs and goals.

Techniques in Hypnosis for Quitting Smoking or Vaping

Hypnotherapy can be a highly effective method for individuals looking to quit smoking or vaping by addressing the psychological and behavioral aspects of addiction. Here are techniques commonly used in hypnotherapy to help individuals quit smoking or vaping:

1. Motivation Enhancement: Hypnopractitioners work with individuals to enhance their motivation to quit. By tapping into their intrinsic desires for a healthier life, they can create a strong foundation for change.

- *Example Script:* "Imagine all the benefits of a smoke-free life – improved health, increased energy, and more freedom. Let these motivations fuel your commitment to quitting."

2. Identifying Triggers: Hypnotherapy helps individuals identify the triggers that prompt them to smoke or vape. By recognizing these triggers, clients can develop strategies to avoid or cope with them.

- *Example Script:* "Think about the situations, emotions, or stressors that lead you to smoke or vape. Becoming aware of these triggers is the first step to regaining control."

3. Visualization of Health: Guided imagery can assist clients in visualizing their improved health and well-being after quitting. This technique reinforces the positive outcomes of quitting.

- *Example Script:* "Imagine your body healing and rejuvenating with each smoke-free day. See yourself breathing deeply, feeling vitality returning to every cell."

4. Breaking Associations: Hypnopractitioners help individuals break the associations between smoking or vaping and pleasurable activities. This includes shifting the perception of smoking as a reward.

- *Example Script:* "Replace the old association with a healthier one. Whenever you think of smoking or vaping, visualize a more enjoyable and fulfilling alternative."

5. Craving Management: Hypnosis provides individuals with tools to manage cravings when they arise. Techniques like self-affirmations can be used to reinforce the commitment to quit.

- *Example Script:* "When a craving hits, repeat to yourself: 'I am in control. I am stronger than this craving.' You have the power to overcome it."

6. Stress Reduction: Stress is a common trigger for smoking or vaping. Hypnotherapy teaches relaxation techniques to manage stress effectively without turning to nicotine.

- *Example Script:* "Picture a place of absolute calm and serenity. Whenever stress arises, you can mentally transport yourself to this peaceful haven."

7. Reinforcing Self-Control: Hypnopractitioners help individuals strengthen their sense of self-control and willpower. Self-hypnosis can be used to boost confidence in resisting the urge to smoke or vape.

- *Example Script:* "You possess an unshakable willpower to choose health and well-being over addiction. Your inner strength grows with each smoke-free moment."

8. Future Pacing: Visualizing a smoke-free future can provide motivation and reinforce the commitment to quitting.

- *Example Script:* "Imagine yourself in the future, enjoying a smoke-free life. Feel the pride and freedom of your success. This is your reality."

9. Post-Quit Support: Hypnotherapy can provide ongoing support after quitting to address potential relapse triggers and maintain a smoke-free or vape-free lifestyle.

- *Example Script:* "You have quit smoking or vaping, and your journey continues. We will work together to ensure your success is permanent."

10. Personalized Approach: Effective hypnotherapy for quitting smoking or vaping is tailored to the individual's unique triggers, habits, and motivations. A skilled hypnopractitioner customizes the approach to meet the client's specific needs.

These techniques, when integrated into a personalized hypnotherapy program, can significantly increase the chances of successfully quitting smoking or vaping. It's essential to work with a trained hypnopractitioner who can provide guidance and support throughout the process, helping individuals break free from the grip of nicotine addiction and embrace a healthier, smoke-free life.

Techniques in Hypnosis for Self-Doubt and Limiting Beliefs

Hypnotherapy is a powerful approach for addressing self-doubt and limiting beliefs that hold individuals back from reaching their full potential. By accessing the subconscious mind, hypnosis can help reprogram negative thought patterns and replace them with empowering beliefs. Here are some effective techniques commonly used in hypnotherapy to overcome self-doubt and limiting beliefs:

1. Positive Affirmations: Hypnopractitioners use positive affirmations to counteract negative self-talk. By repeating affirmations during hypnosis, individuals can gradually shift their self-perception and beliefs.

- *Example Affirmations:* "I am confident and capable." "I believe in myself and my abilities." "I am deserving of success and happiness."

2. Visualization: Guided imagery is employed to help individuals visualize themselves as confident and successful. This technique can create a mental blueprint for a positive self-image.

- *Visualization Exercise:* "Close your eyes and picture yourself in a situation where self-doubt typically arises. See yourself handling it with confidence and ease. Imagine the positive outcomes."

3. Regression Therapy: Hypnotherapy can uncover the root causes of self-doubt and limiting beliefs by exploring past experiences or traumas. Once identified, these experiences can be reframed and healed.

- *Regression Script:* "Allow yourself to drift back in time to a moment when you first felt self-doubt or encountered a limiting belief. We will work on healing that memory and releasing its hold on you."

4. Cognitive Restructuring: This technique involves identifying and challenging negative thought patterns. Hypnotherapy can help individuals reframe these thoughts into more positive and empowering beliefs.

- *Cognitive Restructuring Script:* "Become aware of any negative thoughts about yourself. Now, let's examine them together and transform them into thoughts that support your confidence and self-worth."

5. Anchoring Confidence: Hypnopractitioners assist clients in creating anchors (physical or mental cues) associated with feelings of confidence and self-assurance. These anchors can be activated when self-doubt arises.

- *Anchoring Technique:* "Think of a moment when you felt extremely confident. As you recall that moment, touch your thumb and forefinger together. This anchor will remind you of your inner strength."

6. Self-Esteem Building: Hypnotherapy helps individuals develop a healthier self-esteem by addressing the underlying causes of low self-worth and fostering self-acceptance.

- *Self-Esteem Script:* "You are a unique and valuable individual. Embrace your worthiness and accept yourself unconditionally, just as you are."

7. Future Pacing: Visualizing a future where self-doubt and limiting beliefs no longer have power can provide motivation and reinforce the commitment to change.

- *Future Pacing Exercise:* "Imagine yourself in the future, living a life free from self-doubt and limiting beliefs. Feel the confidence and success that comes with this transformation."

8. Post-Hypnotic Suggestions: Hypnopractitioners provide clients with post-hypnotic suggestions that continue to reinforce positive beliefs and behaviors even outside of hypnosis sessions.

- *Post-Hypnotic Suggestion:* "After this session, you will find that your self-doubt diminishes, and your self-confidence grows stronger with each passing day."

9. Self-Compassion: Hypnotherapy encourages individuals to cultivate self-compassion and treat themselves with kindness and understanding, reducing self-criticism.

- *Self-Compassion Affirmation:* "I am gentle with myself. I recognize that self-doubt is a part of being human, and I choose to be kind to myself."

10. Goal Achievement: Hypnotherapy can be used to set and reinforce positive, achievable goals that build confidence and counteract limiting beliefs.

- *Goal Achievement Script:* "Visualize yourself accomplishing your goals one step at a time. See the progress you make, and believe in your ability to achieve what you desire."

These techniques, when integrated into a hypnotherapy program, can empower individuals to overcome self-doubt and limiting beliefs, enabling them to reach their full potential and live more fulfilling lives. It's important to work with a skilled hypnopractitioner who can tailor the approach to the individual's specific needs and provide guidance and support throughout the process.

Techniques in Hypnosis for Improved Concentration

Hypnotherapy offers valuable techniques for enhancing concentration and focus by tapping into the power of the subconscious mind. Whether you struggle with scattered thoughts, distractions, or a wandering mind, these techniques can help you sharpen your concentration abilities:

1. Deep Relaxation: Hypnotherapy often begins with inducing a state of deep relaxation. When the mind and body are relaxed, it's easier to concentrate without the interference of stress and tension.

- *Relaxation Script:* "Imagine a wave of calmness washing over you, from the top of your head to the tips of your toes. Feel the tension melting away, leaving you in a state of complete relaxation."

2. Visualization: Hypnotherapy uses visualization techniques to create mental images that enhance concentration. Visualizing a focused and productive state of mind can make it easier to achieve.

- *Visualization Exercise:* "Picture yourself in a serene library, surrounded by books and a peaceful atmosphere. As you focus on your work, feel the sense of concentration and clarity growing stronger."

3. Positive Affirmations: Affirmations can reinforce the belief in your ability to concentrate. By repeating positive statements, you can boost your confidence and motivation for focused attention.

- *Affirmation Example:* "I am fully capable of concentrating on the task at hand. My mind is clear, and my focus is unwavering."

4. Anchoring Techniques: Creating anchors, such as a specific touch or gesture, can help trigger a state of heightened concentration when needed.

- *Anchoring Exercise:* "Touch your index finger and thumb together as you enter a state of deep concentration. This anchor will remind you to maintain focus whenever you use it."

5. Mindfulness and Present-Moment Awareness: Hypnotherapy encourages mindfulness, which involves being fully present in the moment. This practice can train your mind to stay focused on the task at hand.

- *Mindfulness Script:* "In this moment, bring your full attention to your breath. Notice each inhale and exhale, letting go of any distractions. This practice sharpens your ability to stay present."

6. Eliminating Distractions: Hypnotherapy can help individuals identify and address specific distractions that hinder concentration. Strategies for managing and minimizing distractions are discussed.

- *Distraction Management:* "Think about the distractions that often interfere with your focus. We will work on strategies to eliminate or reduce these distractions in your daily life."

7. Goal Setting: Setting clear and achievable goals with the help of hypnotherapy can provide direction and motivation, making it easier to maintain concentration.

- *Goal-Setting Exercise:* "Visualize your goals and the steps required to achieve them. This clear sense of purpose will drive your concentration and productivity."

8. Memory Enhancement: Memory exercises during hypnotherapy can improve cognitive functions related to concentration. A sharper memory can aid in retaining information and staying engaged.

- *Memory Enhancement:* "Picture a memory palace where you store important information. This technique enhances your memory and keeps your mind engaged."

9. Stress Reduction: Reducing stress and anxiety through hypnotherapy is essential for improving concentration. A calm mind is more receptive to focusing on tasks.

- *Stress Reduction Script:* "Imagine a serene garden where you release all stress and worry. As you let go of tension, your mind becomes clear and ready to concentrate."

10. Post-Hypnotic Suggestions: Hypnotherapy can provide post-hypnotic suggestions that reinforce improved concentration in daily life.

- *Post-Hypnotic Suggestion:* "After this session, you will find that your concentration has improved significantly. You naturally maintain focus on your tasks with ease."

These techniques, when incorporated into a hypnotherapy program, can empower individuals to boost their concentration and overcome common challenges related to distraction and scattered thinking. Working with a skilled hypnopractitioner who tailors the approach to your specific needs can help you achieve lasting improvements in concentration and focus.

Techniques in Hypnosis for Pain Management

Hypnotherapy offers effective techniques for managing and even alleviating pain through the power of the mind-body connection. While hypnosis does not replace medical treatment, it can be used as a complementary approach to reduce pain perception and improve overall well-being. Here are some techniques commonly used in hypnotherapy for pain management:

1. Deep Relaxation: Hypnotherapy often begins with inducing a state of deep relaxation. This relaxation helps reduce tension, stress, and anxiety, which can exacerbate pain.

- *Relaxation Script:* "Imagine a wave of warmth and relaxation flowing through your body, soothing every muscle. Feel the tension melting away, leaving you in a state of profound calm."

2. Distraction: Hypnosis can redirect your focus away from the pain sensations. By engaging your mind in positive and absorbing imagery, the perception of pain can diminish.

- *Distraction Technique:* "Visualize a serene beach or a peaceful forest. Explore the details of this place, the colors, sounds, and sensations. As you immerse yourself in this mental escape, notice the pain receding."

3. Imagery and Visualization: Guided imagery techniques in hypnotherapy can help individuals visualize their pain as a physical object that can be manipulated or transformed.

- *Imagery Exercise:* "Picture your pain as a cloud of dark smoke. Now, imagine a gentle breeze blowing that smoke away, leaving behind a clear and pain-free space."

4. Altering Pain Sensations: Hypnosis can modify how you perceive pain sensations. By suggesting that pain feels different or less intense, it becomes more manageable.

- *Suggestion Technique:* "Imagine the sensation of warmth or coolness spreading through the area of pain. Feel how this new sensation replaces the pain, making it more bearable."

5. Time Distortion: Hypnotherapy can create a sense of time distortion, making pain feel shorter or less continuous.

- *Time Distortion Exercise:* "As you focus on your breath, notice that time seems to pass more quickly. The pain comes in short, manageable bursts, and the intervals of relief become longer."

6. Pain Gate Control: Hypnosis can influence the gate control theory of pain perception. By suggesting that the "pain gate" is closing, it can reduce the intensity of pain signals.

- *Pain Gate Control Script:* "Imagine a gate in your mind that controls the pain signals. As you visualize it closing, feel the pain diminishing and your comfort increasing."

7. Mindfulness: Hypnotherapy encourages mindfulness, which involves non-judgmental awareness of pain sensations. This practice can help individuals cope with pain more effectively.

- *Mindfulness Exercise:* "Bring your attention to the sensations of pain without judgment. Observe the pain as if you are an impartial observer. This perspective can reduce suffering."

8. Self-Hypnosis for Pain Control: Hypnotherapy teaches self-hypnosis techniques so individuals can manage pain on their own when needed.

- *Self-Hypnosis Method:* "Practice self-hypnosis regularly. When pain arises, use self-hypnosis to apply the techniques you've learned and regain control over your comfort."

9. Post-Hypnotic Suggestions: Hypnotherapy provides post-hypnotic suggestions that continue to reduce pain perception even after the session ends.

- *Post-Hypnotic Suggestion:* "After this session, you will find that your ability to manage and reduce pain has improved. You will naturally apply these techniques when needed."

10. Pain Coping Strategies: Hypnotherapy can help individuals develop effective pain coping strategies, such as positive self-talk and relaxation techniques, to use in daily life.

- *Pain Coping Strategy:* "Practice positive self-talk when pain arises. Remind yourself that you have the inner strength to manage this pain, and you are in control of your comfort."

These techniques, when integrated into a hypnotherapy program, can empower individuals to manage pain more effectively, reduce reliance on pain medications, and improve their overall quality of life. It's important to work with a skilled hypnopractitioner who can tailor the approach to the individual's specific pain condition and provide guidance and support throughout the process.

Techniques in Hypnosis for Disease Management and Healing

Hypnotherapy can play a complementary role in disease management and healing by harnessing the mind's power to enhance physical and emotional well-being. While it is not a substitute for medical treatment, hypnotherapy can support individuals in coping with their conditions and promoting the body's natural healing processes. Here are techniques commonly used in hypnotherapy for disease management and healing:

1. Pain Management: Hypnotherapy can help individuals manage pain associated with various diseases, such as chronic pain, fibromyalgia, or cancer-related pain. Techniques for pain reduction and distraction, as mentioned earlier, can be applied.

- *Pain Management Script:* "As you enter a state of relaxation, imagine the pain diminishing. Picture it becoming less intense, allowing you to find comfort and relief."

2. Stress Reduction: Chronic stress can exacerbate many diseases. Hypnotherapy techniques for stress reduction, including relaxation and mindfulness, help individuals manage stress levels effectively.

- *Stress Reduction Exercise:* "Visualize a serene place where you feel completely at ease. Imagine all stress melting away, leaving you with a sense of calm and balance."

3. Immune System Boosting: Hypnosis can suggest positive changes to the immune system. While it cannot directly cure diseases, it can encourage the body to better fight off illnesses.

- *Immune System Script:* "Visualize your immune system a a strong and vigilant guardian. See it actively defending your body against any threats, promoting healing and recovery."

4. Symptom Management: Hypnotherapy helps individuals cope with disease-related symptoms such as nausea, fatigue, or shortness of breath. Techniques like suggestion and imagery can provide relief.

- *Symptom Management Suggestion:* "Imagine a soothing, healing light surrounding the area of discomfort. Feel this light alleviating your symptoms and restoring your well-being."

5. Visualization of Healing: Guided imagery can assist individuals in visualizing their body's healing and recovery from their specific diseases. This can promote a positive mindset.

- *Healing Visualization Exercise:* "Picture your body's cells working together harmoniously to repair and regenerate. See yourself on a path to full health and vitality."

6. Pain Gate Control: As mentioned earlier, hypnotherapy can influence the gate control theory of pain perception, reducing the intensity of pain signals associated with certain diseases.

- *Pain Gate Control Technique:* "Imagine the gate controlling pain in your body. As it closes, the pain lessens, and you experience greater comfort and relief."

7. Coping with Symptoms: Hypnotherapy teaches individuals coping strategies to manage disease-related symptoms, such as positive self-talk, relaxation, and self-hypnosis techniques.

- *Coping Strategy Affirmation:* "In challenging moments, I have the inner resources to manage my symptoms. I am resilient and capable of finding comfort and relief."

8. Emotional Support: Chronic diseases often come with emotional challenges. Hypnotherapy addresses anxiety, depression, and emotional distress by promoting resilience and emotional well-being.

- *Emotional Support Suggestion:* "Visualize yourself as emotionally resilient. Feel your inner strength, capable of facing challenges with a positive mindset and emotional balance."

9. Lifestyle Changes: Hypnotherapy can assist individuals in making positive lifestyle changes, such as adopting healthier eating habits, quitting smoking, or increasing physical activity.

- *Lifestyle Change Suggestion:* "See yourself making healthy choices effortlessly. Your body and mind naturally gravitate towards actions that promote healing and well-being."

10. Post-Hypnotic Suggestions: Hypnotherapy provides post-hypnotic suggestions that continue to support disease management and healing in daily life, reinforcing positive behaviors and attitudes.

- *Post-Hypnotic Healing Suggestion:* "After this session, you will find that your ability to manage your disease and support your healing has improved. You naturally apply these techniques and foster a state of well-being."

These techniques, when integrated into a hypnotherapy program, can empower individuals to cope with their diseases more effectively, reduce the impact of symptoms, and promote healing and well-being. It is crucial to work with a skilled hypnopractitioner who can tailor the approach to the individual's specific disease, needs, and goals while collaborating with their healthcare team for a comprehensive approach to healing.

Techniques in Hypnosis for Healing Past Trauma

Hypnotherapy can be a valuable tool for addressing and healing past trauma by accessing the subconscious mind and helping individuals process and release emotional wounds. Trauma can have a profound impact on mental and emotional well-being, and these techniques can aid in the healing process. Here are some techniques commonly used in hypnotherapy for past trauma:

1. Safe Space Visualization: Hypnotherapy often begins with establishing a safe and comfortable mental space. This safe space serves as a sanctuary where individuals can feel secure and grounded during the healing process.

- *Safe Space Visualization:* "Close your eyes and picture a place where you feel completely safe and at peace. Visualize every detail, and know that you can return to this space whenever you need comfort."

2. Regression Therapy: Hypnotherapy can guide individuals back to the traumatic event in a controlled and supportive environment. This allows them to revisit the past trauma with the perspective and understanding they have now, helping to release associated emotions.

- *Regression Script:* "Allow yourself to drift back to the moment when the trauma occurred. You are safe and protected as we explore this memory, gain insights, and release any emotional burdens."

3. Reframing Traumatic Memories: Hypnotherapy assists individuals in reframing how they perceive and remember traumatic events. By altering the perspective on the past, the emotional impact can be lessened.

- *Reframing Technique:* "See the traumatic event from a different angle. Imagine it as an experience that taught you resilience and strength, rather than defining your worth."

4. Emotional Release: Hypnotherapy provides a safe space to release pent-up emotions associated with trauma, such as anger, sadness, or fear. By acknowledging and releasing these emotions, individuals can find relief.

- *Emotional Release Exercise:* "Allow yourself to express any emotions connected to the trauma. It's okay to cry, scream, or let out any feelings that have been bottled up."

5. Inner Child Healing: Many traumatic experiences originate in childhood. Hypnotherapy can guide individuals to connect with their inner child, offering comfort, support, and healing to that vulnerable part of themselves.

- *Inner Child Healing:* "Imagine yourself as the child you once were during the traumatic event. Offer comfort, love and protection to your inner child, reassuring them that they are safe now."

6. Positive Anchoring: Creating positive anchors during hypnotherapy helps individuals associate feelings of safety and empowerment with specific triggers or situations related to the trauma.

- *Positive Anchoring Technique:* "As you recall the traumatic memory, simultaneously touch your thumb and forefinger. This anchor will remind you of your strength and resilience."

7. Self-Compassion: Hypnotherapy fosters self-compassion and self-acceptance. Individuals are guided to treat themselves with kindness, understanding, and forgiveness as they work through their trauma.

- *Self-Compassion Affirmation:* "I am worthy of love and compassion. I forgive myself for any perceived shortcomings related to the trauma. I am healing and growing."

8. Post-Trauma Reintegration: Hypnotherapy helps individuals reintegrate the healed aspects of themselves back into their identity. This process allows for a more cohesive and positive sense of self.

- *Reintegration Process:* "Integrate the strength, resilience, and wisdom you've gained from healing your trauma into your self-identity. Embrace your newfound wholeness."

9. Confidence and Empowerment: Hypnotherapy can boost self-confidence and empowerment, enabling individuals to move forward with a renewed sense of purpose and self-assuredness.

- *Empowerment Suggestion:* "You possess the inner strength and resilience to face life's challenges with confidence. Trust in your ability to heal and thrive."

10. Self-Hypnosis for Ongoing Healing: Hypnotherapy teaches self-hypnosis techniques so individuals can continue their healing journey independently, whenever needed.

- *Self-Hypnosis for Healing:* "Practice self-hypnosis regularly to maintain your emotional well-being. You have the tools to nurture your healing process."

These techniques, when integrated into a hypnotherapy program, can empower individuals to heal from past trauma, release emotional burdens, and regain a sense of emotional well-being and resilience. It's essential to work with a skilled hypnopractitioner who can provide guidance and support throughout the healing journey, ensuring a safe and transformative experience.

In addition to Hypnotherapy, some other techniques can help overcome past traumas.

The NLP version of EMDR, Eye Movement Integration (EMI), and Emotional Freedom Techniques (EFT) can be extremely effective for Past Trauma Healing

Eye Movement Integration (EMI) and Emotional Freedom Techniques (EFT) are two therapeutic approaches that have gained recognition for their effectiveness in helping individuals heal from past trauma. These techniques provide innovative ways to process traumatic experiences, release emotional distress, and promote healing. Here's how EMI and EFT can be used for past trauma healing:

Eye Movement Integration (EMI):

While EMI can be the subject of its own book, it is a powerful tool, so it is something that I wanted to bring your attention to. EMI is the kinder, gentler NLP version of EMDR. EMI should only be performed by those trained in its use. In the event of an abreaction, it is important to know how to bring the client back to a place of safety. To find out more about EMI, visit www.hypno-mastery.com

Eye Movement Integration, or EMI for short, is a therapy technique mainly used for helping people who've been through trauma or are dealing with PTSD and anxiety-related issues. It's pretty fascinating how it works. Imagine this: by moving your eyes in certain ways – up and down, side to side, in circles – you can actually start to process and come to terms with really tough memories.

Here is typically how a session would be structured:

Assessment: The practitioner begins by assessing the client's traumatic experiences, and identifying specific memories, emotions, and triggers associated with the trauma.

Eye Movements: The client is guided to make specific eye movements while recalling the traumatic memory. These eye movements are thought to stimulate the brain's processing capacity.

Visualization: During the eye movements, the client is prompted to visualize the traumatic memory in a controlled and safe manner. This process can lead to the desensitization of the traumatic content.

Reprocessing: As the client continues the eye movements and visualization, the practitioner helps them reprocess the traumatic memory, allowing it to become integrated into their broader life narrative.

Emotional Release: EMI often leads to the release of intense emotions associated with the trauma. Clients may experience a reduction in the emotional charge of the memory.

Cognitive Shift: EMI can facilitate a cognitive shift, allowing clients to view the traumatic event from a different perspective, often leading to increased understanding and acceptance.

Integration: The goal of EMI is to help clients integrate the traumatic memory into their life story in a way that no longer exerts a debilitating influence.

Emotional Freedom Techniques (EFT):

EFT is a psychological acupressure technique that combines elements of acupressure and acupuncture points. It involves tapping on specific meridian points on the body while focusing on the traumatic memory or emotional distress. EFT is designed to release blocked energy and alleviate emotional and physical symptoms associated with trauma. Here's how EFT works:

Identification: The practitioner and client identify the specific traumatic memory, emotional issue or discomfort that needs addressing.

Setup Statement: The client formulates a setup statement that acknowledges the issue and affirms self-acceptance. For example, "Even though I have this traumatic memory, I deeply and completely accept myself."

Tapping Sequence: The client then taps on specific acupressure points on the body 7-10 times each before moving on to the next point.

While tapping, the client briefly focuses on the traumatic memory or emotional distress.

Here are the common EFT tapping points:

Karate Chop (KC): The side of the hand (the fleshy part on the outside edge of the hand when making a karate chop).

Top of Head (TH): The crown of your head.

Eyebrow (EB): The beginning of the brow, just above and to one side of the nose.

Side of the Eye (SE): On the bone bordering the outside corner of the eye.

Under the Eye (UE): On the bone under the eye, approximately 1 inch below your pupil.

Under the Nose (UN): The area between the nose and the upper lip.

Chin (Ch): The area just below the bottom lip and above the chin.

Collarbone (CB): The junction where the sternum (breastbone), collarbone, and the first rib meet. A common approach is to tap the area about an inch below the junction.

Under the Arm (UA): On the side of the body, about four inches beneath the armpit.

These points are tapped in sequence while focusing on a specific issue and reciting affirmations or reminder phrases. The process is believed to release blockages in the body's energy system and facilitate emotional and physical healing.

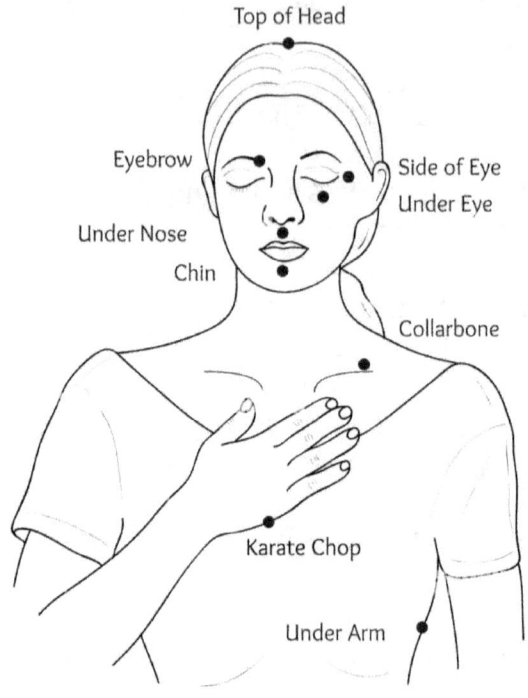

Top of Head

Eyebrow

Side of Eye

Under Eye

Under Nose

Chin

Collarbone

Karate Chop

Under Arm

EFT Tapping Points

Reevaluation: After a few rounds of tapping, the client reevaluates their emotional intensity and physical sensations related to the issue. The goal is to reduce distress.

Repeat as Needed: The tapping sequence is repeated as many times as necessary until the emotional distress significantly diminishes or disappears.

Positive Affirmation: Once the distress is reduced, the client replaces the negative emotional charge with a positive affirmation related to self-acceptance and healing. "Even though I have this _____ I accept myself fully and completely"

EMI (Eye Movement Integration) and EFT (Emotional Freedom Techniques) are both really promising when it comes to healing from past traumas. But, it's important to have a practitioner or practitioner who knows their stuff to lead the way safely and effectively. With the right guidance, these methods can be amazing tools. They help people work through their trauma, dial down the emotional pain, and encourage deep, lasting healing.

Neuro-Linguistic Programming (NLP) Time Techniques for Past Trauma Healing

Neuro-Linguistic Programming (NLP) offers various techniques that can be valuable in healing from past trauma. NLP Time Techniques, in particular, provide innovative ways to revisit and reframe traumatic memories, allowing individuals to release emotional distress and find resolution. Here's how NLP Time Techniques can be used for past trauma healing:

1. Timeline Therapy:

Timeline Therapy is an NLP technique that involves accessing and working with the mental representation of time and memories in one's mind. It allows individuals to revisit past traumatic events, reframe them, and release associated negative emotions. Here's how Timeline Therapy works:

- Accessing the Timeline: The individual is guided to mentally access their timeline, which represents their personal history from the past to the future.
- Identifying Traumatic Events: With the practitioner's guidance, the individual identifies specific traumatic events on their timeline.
- Reframing and Emotional Release: The individual revisits each traumatic event, reframing it by altering the emotional charge and gaining insights. They release negative emotions associated with the trauma, such as anger, sadness, or fear.
- Integration: As the traumatic events are reframed and emotions are released, the individual integrates these transformed memories into their timeline in a way that no longer exerts a negative influence.
- Future Pacing: The individual is guided to envision a positive and empowered future, reinforcing the changes made during the timeline therapy.

2. Change Personal History:

Change Personal History is an NLP technique that allows individuals to rewrite and reframe past traumatic memories to alter their emotional impact and meaning. Here's how Change Personal History works:

- Identifying Target Memories: The individual identifies specific traumatic memories they want to address and change.

- Mental Editing: With the practitioners guidance, the individual mentally edits the traumatic memories, altering the sensory details, emotions, and interpretations.
- Emotional Release: The individual releases any negative emotions associated with the original memories and replaces them with more empowering emotions.
- Reframing and Integration: The revised memories are integrated into the individual's personal history, allowing them to view the past trauma from a new and empowering perspective.
- Positive Anchoring: The practitioner helps the individual anchor positive emotions and resources to the revised memories, making them a source of strength and resilience.

3. Parts Integration:

Parts Integration is an NLP technique that addresses inner conflicts and unresolved issues. It helps individuals integrate conflicting aspects of themselves to find a resolution. Here's how Parts Integration works:

- Identifying Conflicting Parts: The individual identifies conflicting internal parts or aspects related to the trauma, such as the victim part and the empowered part.
- Dialogue and Integration: The practitioner facilitates a dialogue between these parts, allowing them to communicate and understand each other's perspectives.
- Resolution and Integration: Through the dialogue, the conflicting parts can find common ground, resolve the internal conflict, and integrate into a more harmonious and empowered whole.
- Positive Resource Integration: The practitioner helps the individual integrate positive resources and qualities from both parts, strengthening their overall sense of self.

NLP Time Techniques are powerful tools for past trauma healing, as they allow individuals to revisit and reframe traumatic memories, release negative emotions, and create lasting changes in how they perceive and respond to past events. It's important to work with a certified NLP practitioner or practitioner experienced in these techniques to ensure a safe and effective healing process.

Hypnosis Techniques for Children

Hypnotherapy can be an effective and gentle approach for addressing various issues in children, promoting relaxation, and helping them cope with challenges. When working with children, it's essential to create a safe and comfortable environment. Here are some techniques commonly used in hypnotherapy for children:

1. Imaginative Storytelling: Children have vivid imaginations, and using storytelling is a powerful way to engage them in hypnotherapy. The practitioner crafts a story that incorporates relaxation and positive suggestions.

- *Example Story:* "Imagine you are floating on a fluffy cloud, feeling so light and relaxed. As you float, you meet a friendly dragon who tells you that you are brave and strong."

2. Creative Visualization: Children often respond well to visualizations that involve their favorite activities or characters. These visualizations can promote relaxation and positive feelings.

- *Visualization Exercise:* "Close your eyes and imagine you are in your favorite place, like a magical forest or a sunny beach. What do you see, hear, and feel in this special place?"

3. Guided Breathing: Teaching children deep breathing techniques can help them manage stress and anxiety. Simple guided breathing exercises can be incorporated into sessions.

- *Guided Breathing:* "Take a deep breath in, like you are smelling a flower, and then blow it out gently, like you are blowing out birthday candles. Let's do it together."

4. Playful Hypnosis: Hypnotherapy for children often involves playful language and activities that resonate with their interests. Using toys, puppets, or games can make the process enjoyable.

- *Playful Hypnosis Activity:* "Let's use this magic wand (or puppet) to help you relax. When I tap your shoulder with it, you'll feel more and more relaxed, like a sleepy teddy bear."

5. Positive Affirmations: Encouraging children to repeat positive affirmations can boost their self-esteem and confidence.

- *Positive Affirmation:* "Say, 'I am brave and strong,' like a superhero. You are amazing, and you can do anything you set your mind to!"

6. Progressive Muscle Relaxation: Children can benefit from learning to relax their bodies. A playful approach to progressive muscle relaxation can help them release tension.

- *Progressive Muscle Relaxation:* "Let's pretend you're a statue. Squeeze your muscles tight like a superhero, and then relax them like a floppy doll. Feel how relaxed and calm you are."

7. Creative Expression: For older children and teenagers, creative expression techniques such as drawing, journaling, or storytelling can help them explore and process their feelings.

- *Creative Journaling:* "Write or draw about how you are feeling today. You can use any colors and shapes you like. This is your special space to express yourself."

8. Post-Hypnotic Suggestions: Like with adults, providing post-hypnotic suggestions to children can reinforce positive behaviors and attitudes outside of the session.

- *Post-Hypnotic Suggestion:* "After our session, you'll feel more confident and calm in challenging situations. You'll remember that you are strong and capable."

9. Guided Imagery for Sleep: Hypnotherapy can help children with sleep difficulties. Guided imagery that takes them on a soothing journey to sleep can be particularly effective.

- *Sleep Visualization:* "Picture yourself in a cozy sleeping bag under a blanket of stars. With each breath, you become sleepier and more relaxed, drifting into a peaceful slumber."

10. Parental Involvement: Involving parents in the process is crucial for children. Parents can support the child's practice of relaxation techniques at home and reinforce positive changes.

- *Parental Involvement:* "Parents, you can help by practicing these relaxation exercises with your child at home. This will create a comforting routine for them."

When working with children, it's essential to adapt the language and techniques to their age and developmental level. The goal is to create a positive and empowering experience that helps children manage their emotions, build resilience, and develop coping strategies for various challenges they may face. A skilled and compassionate hypnopractitioner can tailor the approach to each child's unique needs and interests.

Hypnosis Techniques for General Life Improvement

Hypnotherapy is a versatile tool that can be used to enhance various aspects of life, promote personal growth, and achieve general life improvement. Whether you're looking to boost self-confidence, manage stress, or break unhealthy habits, hypnotherapy can help. Here are techniques commonly used in hypnotherapy for general life improvement:

1. Self-Confidence Boost: Hypnotherapy can help individuals build self-confidence and a positive self-image. This technique involves suggesting empowering beliefs and self-assuredness.

- *Self-Confidence Suggestion:* "You are confident and capable in all that you do. You believe in yourself and your abilities."

2. Stress Reduction: Hypnotherapy techniques for stress reduction can induce deep relaxation, calm the mind, and reduce anxiety levels.

- *Stress Reduction Exercise:* "Imagine a peaceful place where you feel completely relaxed. As you visualize this place, notice how your stress melts away."

3. Goal Setting and Achievement: Hypnotherapy can help individuals set clear goals and stay motivated to achieve them. Techniques involve visualizing success and reinforcing determination.

- *Goal Achievement Visualization:* "See yourself achieving your goals with enthusiasm and determination. You have the focus and drive to make your dreams a reality."

4. Breaking Habits and Addictions: Hypnotherapy is effective for breaking unhealthy habits and addictions by suggesting new behaviors and reinforcing willpower.

- *Habit-Breaking Suggestion:* "You have the strength to overcome [habit] and replace it with healthier choices. You are in control of your actions."

5. Motivation Enhancement: Hypnotherapy can enhance motivation and enthusiasm for tasks and projects, making it easier to stay productive and reach goals.

- *Motivation Enhancement Technique:* "Feel a surge of motivation and excitement as you approach your tasks. You are energized and ready to accomplish your goals."

6. Positive Thinking: Hypnotherapy helps individuals replace negative thought patterns with positive ones. Techniques involve challenging and reframing pessimistic beliefs.

- *Positive Thinking Affirmation:* "You naturally focus on the positive aspects of life. Optimism and positivity are your default mindset."

7. Overcoming Procrastination: Hypnotherapy can address procrastination by suggesting a proactive and productive approach to tasks and responsibilities.

- *Procrastination-Busting Suggestion:* "You are motivated to tackle tasks with enthusiasm and efficiency. Procrastination is a thing of the past."

8. Pain Management: Hypnotherapy can assist individuals in managing pain, whether it's chronic pain or discomfort from an injury. Techniques involve altering pain perception and promoting relaxation.

- *Pain Management Script:* "Imagine a soothing sensation spreading through the area of pain, replacing discomfort with comfort and ease."

9. Time Management: Hypnotherapy can help individuals improve time management skills by suggesting effective planning and organization strategies.

- *Time Management Suggestion:* "You manage your time wisely and prioritize tasks effectively. Your days are well-structured and productive."

10. Positive Self-Talk: Hypnotherapy encourages positive self-talk and inner dialogue. Techniques involve suggesting self-compassion and self-encouragement.

- *Positive Self-Talk Affirmation:* "Your inner dialogue is filled with kindness and encouragement. You believe in yourself and your abilities."

11. Visualization for Success: Hypnotherapy often incorporates visualization exercises that help individuals vividly imagine their desired outcomes and success.

- *Visualization for Success:* "See yourself achieving your goals in great detail. Feel the excitement and fulfillment that success brings."

12. Self-Hypnosis Training: Hypnotherapy teaches individuals self-hypnosis techniques so they can continue to reinforce positive changes independently.

- *Self-Hypnosis for Continual Improvement:* "Practice self-hypnosis regularly to maintain and enhance your personal growth journey. You have the tools to create a better life."

These techniques, when integrated into a hypnotherapy program, can empower individuals to make positive changes, overcome challenges, and enhance their overall quality of life. It's important to work with a skilled hypnopractitioner who can tailor the approach to the individual's specific goals and needs, providing guidance and support throughout the process of general life improvement.

Chapter 10:
Empowering the Self - Self-Hypnosis

Self-hypnosis is a handy tool to have in your personal wellness toolkit. It's something you can do on your own time, it's free, and you can tailor it to exactly what you need at the moment. It's great for calming down, reducing stress, and pumping yourself up with positive vibes. For those who've got the hang of it, it can be a lifesaver for easing anxiety, sharpening focus, or even getting better sleep.

But, and this is a big but, self-hypnosis doesn't usually pack the same punch as seeing a professional hypnotherapist. Think about it like this: doing yoga at home using a video is good for you, sure, but it's not quite the same as having a yoga instructor right there, tailoring the session to your needs, and helping you perfect your poses.

A trained hypnotherapist knows how to dive deep. They can guide you into a deeper trance than you might manage on your own. They're like a tour guide in the world of your subconscious, able to steer the session based on how you're responding right there and then.

More than that, a hypnotherapist can get to the root of bigger, trickier issues. If you're dealing with long-standing phobias, old traumas, or habits that are hard to break, that's where a trained professional can make a big impact on the issue. They create a safe and structured space, which is especially crucial when you're dealing with deep issues.

Don't forget the power of the therapist-client relationship either. Having someone you trust, who's rooting for you and understands the journey you're on, can make all the difference. It's that extra layer of support and insight that you just can't get doing self-hypnosis.

So, while self-hypnosis is fantastic for daily self-care and handling the regular ups and downs of life, when it comes to deeper, more complex stuff, or if you're looking for a really impactful hypnosis experience, you're probably going to get more out of sessions with a qualified hypnotherapist.

Key Elements of Self-Hypnosis

Relaxation: The first step is to relax the body deeply. This can be achieved through deep breathing, progressive muscle relaxation, or visualization techniques.

Concentration: Once relaxed, the focus shifts to achieving a state of concentrated attention. This often involves focusing on a specific thought, mantra, or visualization.

Suggestion: In this state, the individual introduces positive affirmations or suggestions to themselves. These are tailored to their specific goals, such as overcoming anxiety, improving confidence, or changing a habit.

Visualization: Many practitioners use visualization techniques, picturing themselves successfully achieving their goal, which can reinforce the positive messages.

Entering and Exiting: Learning how to gently enter into and come out of the self-hypnotic state is crucial. This usually involves counting down to enter and counting up to exit, or visualizing stepping down into a relaxed state and then stepping back up to full awareness.

Uses of Self-Hypnosis

- Stress Relief: Helps in reducing stress and anxiety.
- Behavior Modification: Useful in breaking bad habits, such as smoking or overeating.
- Pain Management: Can be effective in managing chronic pain.
- Personal Development: Aids in improving self-esteem, motivation, and overall mental well-being.

Advantages

- Control: Individuals have complete control over the process and content.
- Convenience: Can be practiced anytime, anywhere, without the need for external assistance.
- Cost-Effective: A free and accessible tool once the techniques are learned.

Getting Started

- Learning the Technique: It's often helpful to initially learn self-hypnosis from a qualified hypnotherapist or through reputable resources.
- Regular Practice: Like any skill, effectiveness improves with regular practice.
- Setting Realistic Goals: Start with small, achievable goals to experience success and build confidence in the technique.

Self-hypnosis is a versatile and powerful tool that can be tailored to a wide range of personal goals. It's a skill that promotes self-care and can enhance overall mental wellness.

Here is a simple breakdown of using self-hypnosis for stress relief:

Step 1: Preparation

- Choose a Quiet Space: Find a quiet, comfortable place where you won't be disturbed.
- Set the Mood: Dim the lights, and maybe play some soft, calming music if it helps you relax.
- Comfortable Position: Sit or lie down in a position that's comfortable for you.

Step 2: Deep Relaxation

- Deep Breathing: Start with deep, slow breaths. Inhale deeply through your nose, hold for a moment, and exhale slowly through your mouth.
- Muscle Relaxation: Progressively relax each muscle group in your body. Start from your toes, gradually moving up to your head, consciously relaxing each part.

Step 3: Inducing Hypnosis

- Focus Your Attention: Focus on a point in the room or close your eyes and imagine a spot in your mind.
- Use a Hypnotic Induction: Slowly count down from 10 to 1, telling yourself with each count that you're becoming more relaxed and going deeper into a hypnotic state.

Step 4: Deepening the Hypnotic State

- Visualization: Imagine yourself in a place where you feel completely at ease. This could be a real place or an imaginary one. Visualize the details of this place - the sights, sounds, and smells.
- Counting Deeper: Optionally, you can deepen the state by imagining yourself walking down a staircase, counting each step down from 10 to 1, going deeper with each step.

Step 5: Positive Suggestions

- Affirmations: Start introducing positive affirmations related to stress relief. For example, "With every breath, I feel more relaxed" or "I am calm and in control of my feelings."
- Visualize Stress Melting Away: Picture any stress or tension in your body as a color or a substance that is slowly dissolving or being washed away.

Step 6: Anchoring the State

- Create an Anchor: This can be a physical gesture (like touching your thumb and forefinger) or a word that you associate with this state of relaxation. Use this anchor whenever you feel stressed to recall this relaxed state.

Step 7: Returning to Full Awareness

- Counting Up: Slowly count from 1 to 5, telling yourself that with each number, you're becoming more aware and alert.

- Stretch and Move: Gently start moving your fingers and toes, then stretch your body. Open your eyes when you're ready.

Step 8: Reflect

- Take a Moment: Spend a few minutes reflecting on the experience. Notice how you feel in comparison to before the session.
- Journaling: Optionally, keep a journal to record your experiences and any insights you gained.

Tips for Success

- Stay Patient: Don't worry if it takes time to get the hang of it. Self-hypnosis is a skill that improves with practice.
- Personalize Your Script: Over time, create a script that resonates best with you and addresses your specific stressors.

Chapter 11:
The Future of Hypnosis

The future of hypnotherapy across various fields holds exciting possibilities. As research deepens and awareness grows, its integration and effectiveness in areas like medicine, psychology, addiction treatment, trauma therapy, and entertainment are expected to expand.

Medical Field

In the medical arena, hypnotherapy's role is increasingly being recognized as a valuable complementary treatment. Its application in pain management is particularly promising. Chronic pain conditions, often resistant to conventional treatments, can be alleviated through hypnotherapy, which works by altering the patient's perception of pain. For childbirth, hypnotherapy is being explored as a method to reduce anxiety and pain, offering a natural alternative or supplement to pain relief medications.

Pain Management and Chronic Conditions

Chronic pain conditions, which are often challenging to manage through conventional treatments, are seeing promising results with hypnotherapy. By altering a patient's perception of pain, hypnotherapy can provide significant relief and improve the quality of life for those suffering from persistent pain. In childbirth, hypnotherapy is increasingly explored as a means to reduce anxiety and manage pain, offering a natural complement or alternative to traditional pain relief methods.

Gastrointestinal Disorders

Hypnotherapy has shown notable efficacy in treating gastrointestinal disorders, such as Irritable Bowel Syndrome (IBS). By improving symptoms and the overall quality of life for patients with IBS, hypnotherapy offers a non-pharmacological approach to managing this complex condition.

Surgical Applications

In surgical settings, hypnotherapy is utilized for preoperative preparation, reducing patient anxiety, and aiding in pain control post-surgery. This approach not only enhances patient comfort but can also contribute to quicker recovery times and reduced reliance on pain medication.

Cancer Treatment

In the context of cancer treatment, hypnotherapy is emerging as a supportive tool to help patients cope with the emotional and psychological impact of cancer diagnosis and treatment. It can aid in managing treatment-related side effects like nausea and fatigue, improve sleep patterns, and provide emotional support through the healing process. The understanding that every disease has an emotional root is particularly pertinent in cancer care, where the psychological well-being of the patient is as crucial as the physical treatment.

Dental Care

Dental care is another field where hypnotherapy is making inroads. It's being used to alleviate dental anxiety, a significant barrier preventing many individuals from seeking necessary dental care. Hypnotherapy can help patients overcome fear, reduce anxiety during procedures, and even manage pain, leading to more positive dental experiences and outcomes.

The Emotional Root of Diseases

The concept that every disease has an emotional root underscores the holistic approach of hypnotherapy. By addressing the psychological and emotional aspects of physical ailments, hypnotherapy can contribute to overall healing and wellness. This mind-body connection is fundamental to the practice of hypnotherapy and is a key factor in its effectiveness across a wide range of medical applications.

Psychology

In psychology, hypnotherapy's integration with traditional therapeutic methods is a key area of development. Its ability to access the subconscious mind makes it a powerful tool for addressing deep-seated issues like phobias, anxiety, and depression. Future advancements may involve combining hypnotherapy with Cognitive Behavioral Therapy (CBT) and other modalities to create more comprehensive treatment plans.

Moreover, hypnotherapy is being explored in treating sleep disorders, stress management, and improving performance, whether in academics, sports, or personal life. Its potential to enhance mindfulness and overall mental well-being signifies a growing role in the realm of psychological therapies.

Addiction Treatment

Hypnotherapy's role in addiction treatment is becoming more prominent. It offers a non-pharmacological approach to breaking the cycle of addiction, addressing both the physical and psychological aspects. By helping modify addictive behaviors and addressing underlying emotional triggers, hypnotherapy can complement traditional treatments like counseling and medication. Its use in smoking cessation and alcohol dependence has shown encouraging results, opening avenues for its application in other forms of addiction.

Trauma Treatment

In trauma therapy, hypnotherapy's gentle approach to accessing and processing traumatic memories makes it a valuable tool. Its potential in dissociating traumatic experiences and reframing them in a safe environment is gaining attention. Combining hypnotherapy with established trauma therapies like EMDR (Eye Movement Desensitization and Reprocessing) could offer more holistic care for those suffering from PTSD and other trauma-related conditions.

Entertainment

The entertainment industry's use of hypnosis, primarily through stage shows, continues to evolve. The fascination and intrigue surrounding hypnotherapy provide a unique entertainment experience. The future might see the integration of hypnotherapy with emerging technologies like virtual reality, offering immersive and interactive experiences. This could open up new avenues for performance art and audience engagement, taking stage hypnosis to new heights.

Chapter 12:
Ethical and Legal Considerations

Ethical and legal considerations are foundational aspects of the practice of hypnosis, ensuring the responsible, safe, and respectful use of this powerful therapeutic tool. In this chapter, we delve deeper into the importance of ethical practice and explore the legal framework that governs hypnotherapy, recognizing that adherence to these principles is crucial for both clients and practitioners.

Ensuring Ethical Practice:

Ethical practice in hypnotherapy is essential to maintain trust, protect clients' well-being, and uphold the integrity of the profession. Here, we expand on key principles of ethical practice in hypnosis:

> **Informed Consent:** Informed consent goes beyond obtaining a signature on a form. It involves a comprehensive discussion with the client, ensuring they understand the nature of hypnotherapy, its purpose, potential risks, and benefits. The client must provide voluntary and informed consent before any hypnosis session.
>
> - *Example:* Before starting a session, a hypnotherapist discusses the goals, processes, and potential outcomes of hypnotherapy with the client. They answer any questions to ensure the client's full understanding.

Client Autonomy: Respecting client autonomy is fundamental. Clients have the right to make decisions about their treatment, including the choice to discontinue sessions or refuse specific suggestions. Hypnotherapists should never impose their beliefs or judgments on clients.

- *Example:* If a client decides to terminate a session due to discomfort, the hypnotherapist respects their decision and discusses alternative approaches.

Confidentiality: Hypnotherapists must maintain strict confidentiality regarding all client information and disclosures. Exceptions to confidentiality should be clearly communicated and comply with legal and ethical obligations.

- *Example:* A hypnotherapist refrains from discussing a client's case with anyone, including friends or family, without the client's explicit consent.

Competence: Hypnotherapists should have appropriate training and qualifications in hypnotherapy. Continuous professional development and supervision are essential to ensure ongoing competency.

- *Example:* A hypnotherapist regularly participates in advanced training courses and receives supervision to enhance their skills and knowledge.

Avoiding Harm: The primary responsibility of a hypnotherapist is to promote the well-being of the client. Hypnosis should never be used to exploit, manipulate, or harm individuals for personal gain or any other reason.

- *Example:* A hypnotherapist is vigilant in monitoring the emotional well-being of their clients and adjusts the therapeutic approach as needed to ensure a safe and supportive environment.

Client Welfare: The focus of hypnotherapy should always be the welfare and benefit of the client. Hypnotherapists should avoid conflicts of interest that may compromise this focus, such as financial gain.

- *Example:* A hypnotherapist refrains from recommending unnecessary sessions to maximize profits and instead suggests the most appropriate and cost-effective treatment plan.

Respect for Diversity: Hypnotherapists should respect the cultural, religious, and individual beliefs of their clients. They must be adaptable and sensitive, tailoring their approach to accommodate diverse backgrounds and perspectives.

- *Example:* A hypnotherapist is aware of cultural nuances and avoids using language or symbols that may be offensive or insensitive to a client's cultural or religious beliefs.

Understanding the Legal Framework:

Navigating the legal landscape is essential for hypnotherapists to practice within the boundaries of the law and uphold their ethical responsibilities. While legal regulations may vary by jurisdiction, here are common legal considerations:

Licensing and Certification: Researching and complying with local licensing requirements is essential. In some areas, hypnotherapists may need specific licenses or certifications to practice legally.

- *Example:* To practice hypnotherapy in Florida, a hypnotist can not work on any issue that would require a license in a medical field. You can not work with someone for pain, anxiety, depression or any other diagnosable condition unless you are a doctor. (it's a stupid law, but it is the law)

Scope of Practice: Hypnotherapists should operate within the scope of their training and expertise. Offering services beyond one's competence can lead to legal repercussions.

- *Example:* A hypnotherapist with expertise in smoking cessation does not attempt to provide therapy for severe psychological disorders outside their area of competence.

Informed Consent Documentation: Maintaining detailed records of informed consent forms signed by clients is advisable. These documents should outline the nature of hypnotherapy, its purpose, potential risks, and benefits.

- *Example:* A hypnotherapist keeps thorough records of informed consent forms, including any specific client concerns or requests discussed during the consent process.

Confidentiality: Legal regulations often mandate strict confidentiality of client information. Hypnotherapists must ensure that their practices comply with relevant privacy laws.

- *Example:* A hypnotherapist stores client records securely, and access to client information is restricted to authorized personnel only.

Liability Insurance: Hypnotherapists may consider obtaining professional liability insurance to protect themselves in case of legal claims or disputes related to their practice.

- *Example:* A hypnotherapist secures liability insurance to provide financial protection in the event of a legal complaint by a client.

Child and Vulnerable Adult Protection: When working with children or vulnerable adults, hypnotherapists should adhere to additional legal safeguards and reporting requirements.

- *Example:* A hypnotherapist follows mandatory reporting procedures if they suspect abuse or neglect of a child they are working with during sessions.

Advertising and Marketing: Truth in advertising regulations should be followed, and hypnotherapists should avoid making false or misleading claims about their services in marketing materials.

- *Example:* A hypnotherapist ensures that all advertising materials accurately represent the services offered and the benefits clients can expect.

Ethical Codes of Conduct: Many professional hypnotherapy organizations have established ethical codes of conduct that practitioners should follow to maintain legal and ethical standards.

- *Example:* A hypnotherapist is a member of a recognized professional organization and adheres to its ethical code, which provides guidance on legal and ethical best practices.

Emergency Procedures: Having clear emergency procedures in place, including contact information for relevant authorities or medical professionals, is crucial to handle unexpected situations during sessions.

- *Example:* A hypnotherapist is prepared to contact emergency services if a client experiences a medical emergency or severe psychological distress during a session.

Complaint Resolution: Hypnotherapists should have mechanisms for addressing client complaints and disputes, which may include mediation or legal processes.

- *Example:* A hypnotherapist has a documented procedure for addressing client complaints, with steps to investigate and resolve issues promptly and professionally.

Ethical and legal considerations are integral to the practice of hypnotherapy. By upholding ethical principles and adhering to legal requirements, hypnotherapists not only provide effective and safe services but also protect the rights and well

Chapter 13
The Hypnotherapy Interview

Conducting a hypnotherapy interview is one of the most important parts of the therapeutic process. It provides essential insights into the client's issues, goals, and suitability for hypnotherapy. We need to know in detail what changes the client wants to make. Here's a guide on how to conduct an effective hypnotherapy interview:

Introduction

- Explain the Process: Briefly outline what the interview will involve and the purpose it serves.

    "Welcome to your initial hypnotherapy session. Before we begin, I'd like to briefly explain what we'll be doing today and why it's important. This initial meeting is what we call a 'discovery session.' Our main goal today is to understand more about you, the challenges you're facing, and what you hope to achieve through hypnotherapy.

    During our time together, I'll ask you a series of questions about your current situation, your health history, any past treatments you've had, and your overall goals for therapy. This is also a great opportunity for you to ask any questions you might have and to express any concerns or preferences regarding the therapy process.

The information you share will help me tailor our future sessions to meet your specific needs and objectives. It's important for me to understand not just the issues you're facing, but also your background and your perspective on them. This helps in creating a therapy plan that's as effective and comfortable for you as possible.

Please remember that everything discussed in these sessions is strictly confidential, and the purpose of these questions is purely to aid in your treatment. Your comfort and trust are paramount, so feel free to share as much or as little as you're comfortable with, and we can proceed at a pace that works best for you.

Does that make sense? Do you have any questions before we begin?"

Building Rapport

- Active Listening: Show genuine interest in what the client says, using non-verbal cues like nodding and maintaining eye contact.
- Empathy: Demonstrate understanding and empathy towards the client's experiences and emotions.

Gathering Information

Asking About the Issue: Start by gently inquiring about what brought them to seek hypnotherapy. Example: "I'm interested to know what brings you to hypnotherapy. Could you share the specific issue or challenge you'd like to address?"

Listening and Acknowledging:

- Active Listening: Pay close attention to their response, showing empathy and understanding.
- Acknowledgement: Validate their feelings and experiences. Example: "It sounds like you've been dealing with a lot of stress, and that's been really challenging for you."

Reframing Into a Positive Statement:

- Identify the Desired Outcome: Focus on what the client wants to achieve rather than what they want to avoid or eliminate. Example: "You mentioned feeling stressed. Let's talk about how we can work towards a state of calmness and control. What would feeling more relaxed and in control look like for you?"
- Highlighting Strengths and Resources: Emphasize the client's strengths or past successes. Example: "You've shown a lot of resilience by managing this far and seeking help. That's a strong foundation we can build on. What are some moments or strategies in the past that have helped you feel more relaxed?"
- Future-Oriented Language: Shift the focus to future possibilities and positive change. Example: "As we work together, we'll explore ways to enhance your ability to cope with stress. Imagine a time in the future when you've successfully managed these feelings. What does that future look like for you?"

Assessing Hypnotherapy Suitability

Assessing the suitability of hypnotherapy for a client is a crucial step in the process. It involves evaluating whether hypnotherapy and/or NLP is the appropriate modality to address the client's specific issues and goals. Here's a detailed approach to this assessment:

1. Understanding Client's Issues and Goals

- Detailed Inquiry: Ask specific questions to understand the nature and severity of the client's issues. Example: "Can you describe how this issue affects your daily life?"
- Goal Setting: Determine what the client hopes to achieve through hypnotherapy. Example: "What specific changes or improvements are you looking to make through our sessions?"

2. Evaluating Psychological and Medical History

- Mental Health: Inquire about any past or present mental health diagnoses or treatments. Example: "Have you ever been diagnosed with a mental health condition or sought counseling before?"
- Physical Health: Discuss any physical health conditions that might impact the hypnotherapy process. Example: "Do you have any ongoing medical conditions or are you taking any medications that we should be aware of?"

3. Considering Hypnotherapy Contraindications

- Identifying Red Flags: Be vigilant for conditions where hypnotherapy might be contraindicated, such as severe mental health disorders. Example: "Given your history of schizophrenia, we need to consider how hypnotherapy might interact with your condition and treatment plan."
- Client Safety: Ensure that hypnotherapy will not pose any risk to the client's physical or mental well-being.

4. Assessing Motivation and Expectations

- Client's Motivation: Gauge the client's readiness and willingness to engage in the hypnotherapy process. Example: "How committed are you to making changes in your life through this therapy?"
- Realistic Expectations: Ensure that the client has realistic and achievable expectations. Example: "While hypnotherapy can be very effective for stress management, it's not an instant cure. It's a collaborative process requiring active participation."

5. Understanding Previous Therapeutic Experiences

- Past Therapies: Discuss any previous therapies and their outcomes. This can provide insight into what has or hasn't worked in the past.
- Client's Response to Hypnosis: If the client has previously experienced hypnosis, ask about their reactions and responses to it. Example: "Have you undergone hypnosis before, and if so, how did you find the experience?"

6. Client's Beliefs and Perceptions about Hypnosis

- Perceptions of Hypnosis: Understanding the client's beliefs about hypnosis can be crucial. Misconceptions or skepticism can affect the therapeutic outcome. Example: "What are your thoughts about hypnosis? Do you have any concerns or misconceptions about it?"

7. Discussing Commitment and Compliance

- Time and Effort: Discuss the commitment required for effective hypnotherapy, including frequency of sessions and at-home practices. Example: "Are you able to commit to regular sessions and practice some techniques at home?"

8. Making an Informed Decision

- Collaborative Decision-Making: Based on the information gathered, collaboratively decide with the client whether hypnotherapy is a suitable choice.
- Referral If Necessary: If hypnotherapy isn't suitable, provide referrals to other types of therapies or specialists.

9. Documenting the Assessment

- Record Keeping: Document all aspects of the assessment for reference in future sessions and for ongoing treatment planning.

By thoroughly assessing the suitability of hypnotherapy, therapists can ensure that they provide the most appropriate and effective treatment for their clients, while also setting a clear and realistic framework for the therapeutic journey ahead.

Closing the Hypnotherapy Interview

The closing phase of a hypnotherapy interview is as crucial as the initial stages. It involves summarizing the key points discussed, outlining the next steps, and addressing any final questions or clarifications. Here's how to effectively close the interview:

Summarizing Key Points

- Recap of Discussion: Review the main issues and goals that emerged during the interview. Example: "Today we discussed your goal to manage stress better and the challenges you've been facing with anxiety."
- Acknowledging Insights: Recognize any insights or significant moments from the session. Example: "It was insightful to learn how your stress is linked to your work environment."
- Reinforcing Goals: Reiterate the client's stated goals to ensure mutual understanding. Example: "So, our primary focus will be on developing strategies to help you cope with stress more effectively."

Outlining Next Steps

- Therapy Plan Overview: Give a brief overview of what the client can expect in future sessions. Example: "In our upcoming sessions, we'll start with some relaxation techniques and work towards identifying triggers for your stress."

- Frequency and Duration: Discuss the proposed frequency and duration of the sessions. Example: "I recommend we meet weekly for 50-minute sessions to start with."
- Home Practice: If applicable, mention any practices or activities the client might engage in between sessions. Example: "I'll also provide you with some simple breathing exercises to practice at home."

Questions and Clarifications

- Inviting Questions: Encourage the client to ask any questions they may have. Example: "Do you have any questions or concerns about what we've discussed or about hypnotherapy in general?"
- Addressing Uncertainties: Take time to clarify any points the client is unsure about. This could be about the therapy process, techniques used, or expected outcomes.
- Reassuring Client: Provide reassurance to help the client feel comfortable and confident moving forward. Example: "It's normal to feel a bit uncertain at this stage, but I'm here to guide you through each step of the process."

Closing Remarks

- Positive Note: End the session on a positive and encouraging note. Example: "I'm looking forward to working with you and helping you achieve your goals."
- Gratitude: Thank the client for their openness and trust. Example: "Thank you for sharing your experiences with me today. It's a significant first step."

Post-Interview Actions

- Documentation: After the client leaves, document the key points of the interview for future reference.
- Planning: Begin planning the first therapy session based on the goals and information gathered during the interview.

By effectively closing the interview, you not only ensure that the client leaves with a clear understanding of the therapy process and what to expect but also reinforce their decision to engage i hypnotherapy, fostering a sense of optimism and trust as they embark on their therapeutic journey.

A successful hypnotherapy interview requires a balance of professionalism, empathy, and skilled questioning. It sets the foundation for a trusting therapist-client relationship and paves the way for a personalized and effective hypnotherapy treatmer plan.

Chapter 14
Progressive Relaxation Script

[Begin with a calm and soothing tone.]

"Find a comfortable and quiet place where you can fully relax. now go ahead and, close your eyes. Take a deep breath in and exhale slowly. Let go of any tension or stress you may be feeling."

[Pause for a few seconds to allow the listener to take a few deep breaths.]

"As you continue to breathe deeply and naturally, focus your attention on your body. Start by directing your awareness to your feet. Imagine a warm, comforting light slowly descending upon your feet. Feel the gentle warmth as it envelops your toes and heels. Let go of any tension in your feet, allowing them to become completely relaxed."

[Pause for a moment to allow the listener to focus on their feet.]

"Now, let that soothing light travel up to your ankles. Feel the relaxation spreading through your ankles, releasing any tightness or discomfort. Your ankles are becoming loose and limp."

[Pause again, emphasizing the relaxation in the ankles.]

"As the warmth moves up to your calves, let go of any tension stored there. Your calves are now completely relaxed, like soft, warm putty."

[Pause, allowing the relaxation to deepen in the calves.]

"Allow that comforting light to ascend to your knees, and as it does, feel any remaining tension melting away. Your knees are now pleasantly relaxed."

[Pause, focusing on the relaxation in the knees.]

"The gentle light now flows up to your thighs, soothing and calming every muscle. Your thighs are warm, heavy, and relaxed."

[Pause, emphasizing the relaxation in the thighs.]

"Feel that peaceful light moving up to your hips and pelvic area. Let go of any stress or discomfort you may be holding in this area. Your hips and pelvis are now completely at ease."

[Pause, giving time for the relaxation to deepen.]

"Now, the soothing light continues to rise, enveloping your abdomen and lower back. Release any tension in this area, allowing your abdomen to rise and fall with each relaxed breath

[Pause, emphasizing relaxation in the abdomen and lower back.

"As the warmth travels up to your chest and upper back, feel your chest expanding with each breath. Your heart rate slows, and your chest and upper back are now deeply relaxed."

[Pause, allowing the listener to focus on their chest and upper back.]

"Let that comforting light flow down to your shoulders, arms, and hands. Feel any tightness in your shoulders melt away. You arms and hands are pleasantly heavy and relaxed."

[Pause, emphasizing relaxation in the shoulders, arms, and hands.]

"Now, bring your attention to your neck and throat. Release any tension in this area, allowing your throat to feel open and free."

[Pause, giving time for relaxation in the neck and throat.]

"Finally, let the soothing light rise to your face and head. Feel your facial muscles relaxing. Your jaw is loose, your forehead smooth, and your scalp relaxed."

[Pause, emphasizing relaxation in the face and head.]

Continue with a hypnotic deepener.

Chapter 15
Hypnosis Deepener

It's important to always deepen the trance state. Below is an example of an effective deepener.

[Begin with a calm and reassuring tone.]

"Now that you are in a state of hypnosis, we are going to deeper this experience further, allowing you to access even deeper levels of relaxation in the body and mind. You are safe and in control at all times, and you can trust this process completely."

[Pause for a few seconds to allow the listener to relax further.]

"I want you to imagine yourself in a beautiful, tranquil garden. This garden represents your subconscious mind. Picture it in vivid detail, noticing the colors, the scents, and the sounds around you."

[Pause as the listener visualizes the garden.]

"As you walk deeper into this garden, you notice a staircase. This staircase has exactly 10 steps, and in a moment you will imagine walking down this staircase, and with each step you descend, you will go even deeper into a wonder state of relation The relaxation doubles with each step you take

[Begin counting down with a slow pace, about 3-4 seconds per number.]

"10... Take the first step, feeling your body and mind relaxing further. 9... Going deeper now. 8... Each step takes you closer to a state of profound awareness. 7... Letting go even more. 6... You are descending into a tranquil state of consciousness."

[Pause briefly.]

"5... Halfway there. 4... Your subconscious mind is open and receptive. 3... Deeper still, feeling completely at ease. 2... Almost at the deepest level of relaxation. 1... You are now at the bottom of the staircase, in the deepest state of hypnosis."

[Pause to acknowledge the deepened state of hypnosis.]

"In this deep state of hypnosis, you have access to the inner resources and wisdom of your subconscious mind. You can explore your inner world, find solutions to challenges, and make positive changes."

[Begin suggestion script]

Chapter 16
Smoking or Vaping Cessation Script example.

[After induction and deepener]

[use a more authoritative voice]

"Imagine yourself in a peaceful place, a place where you feel completely at ease and safe. This is your inner sanctuary, a place where you can find comfort and strength."

[Pause as the listener visualizes their inner sanctuary.]

"In this sanctuary, you are surrounded by a warm, healing light. This light represents your inner strength and determination. Fee it filling you with courage and resolve."

[Pause as the listener connects with their inner strength.]

"Now, I want you to visualize your smoking or vaping habit. Picture it as a heavy burden, a weight that you've carried for far too long. Imagine it in vivid detail."

[Pause as the listener visualizes the habit.]

"See yourself holding this burden in your hands. Feel its weight. Now, visualize yourself letting it go. Imagine it slowly floating away from you, disappearing into the distance."

[Pause, emphasizing the act of letting go.]

"As this burden fades away, you feel a profound sense of relief and freedom. You are no longer controlled by this habit. You are in control of your choices and your health."

[Pause for a moment to allow the listener to absorb the sensation of freedom.]

"From this moment forward, you no longer desire to smoke or vape. The thought of smoking or vaping repels you. You are now a non-smoker, a non-vaper, and you are proud of this positive change in your life."

[Pause, reinforcing the positive change.]

"Whenever you feel tempted to smoke or vape, you will remember this moment of liberation. You will choose health and well-being over the old habit. You are strong, and you have the power to stay smoke-free and vape-free."

[Pause, instilling confidence.]

"In a moment, I will count from 1 to 5, and with each number, you will become more alert and awake. When I reach the number 5, you will be fully awake, refreshed, and ready to embrace your smoke-free, vape-free life."

[Begin the awakening process.]

"1... Starting to awaken now. 2... Feeling more alert. 3... Slowly coming back to your full awareness. 4... Almost there, feeling a sense of freedom. 5... You are now fully awake, refreshed, and ready to embrace your smoke-free, vape-free life."

[End the session with a calm and reassuring tone.]

Chapter 17
Weight loss Script Example

[After induction and deepener]

"Today, we are going to work together to help you achieve your weight loss goals. I want you to understand that you already possess the strength and determination needed to make positive changes in your life. As you continue to relax, know that you are taking a significant step towards a healthier, happier, and more confident you."

[Pause, emphasizing the importance of the journey.]

"Visualize yourself in a serene and natural setting. This is your inner sanctuary, a place of tranquility and inner peace. Picture it in vivid detail, paying attention to the beauty of this place, the colors, the fragrances, and the soothing sounds that surround you."

[Pause as the listener visualizes their inner sanctuary.]

"In this sanctuary, you are bathed in a warm, healing light. This light symbolizes your inner strength and resilience. Feel it enveloping you, filling you with confidence, determination, and a sense of profound well-being."

[Pause as the listener connects with their inner strength.]

"Now, let's bring your ideal self into focus. Imagine yourself at your desired weight, feeling vibrant, healthy, and confident. See yourself radiating with energy and self-assuredness. Visualize every detail of this ideal you."

[Pause as the listener visualizes their ideal self.]

"You are already on the path to becoming this remarkable person. Your subconscious mind is your most powerful ally on this journey. It will assist you in making choices that are in alignment with your weight loss goals."

[Pause, emphasizing the profound influence of the subconscious mind.]

"From this moment forward, you have a deep and unshakable desire to make healthy choices. You naturally gravitate towards nourishing foods that support your well-being and vitality. The pleasure of eating healthy nourishes both your body and your soul."

[Pause for a moment to allow the listener to absorb the positive changes.]

"Physical activity and exercise become sources of joy and empowerment in your life. You eagerly engage in activities that invigorate your body and mind, helping you achieve your weight loss goals while strengthening your self-esteem."

[Pause, reinforcing the enjoyment of an active lifestyle.]

"You've released the need to use food as a way to cope with stress or emotions. You have healthier and more constructive ways to manage your feelings. Mindful eating becomes your practice; you savor each bite and listen to your body's signals, stopping when you are satisfied."

[Pause, reinforcing mindful eating habits.]

"Whenever you encounter challenges or setbacks on your journey, you draw upon your resilience and determination. You remind yourself of your goals, your inner strength, and your unwavering commitment to a healthier life."

[Pause, instilling unwavering determination.]

"Each day, as you awaken, you greet the morning with enthusiasm and motivation. You recognize that every day is an opportunity to make choices that align with your vision of a healthier and happier you."

[Pause, emphasizing the daily commitment.]

"In a moment, I will count from 1 to 5, and with each number, you will become more alert and awake. When I reach the number 5, you will be fully awake, refreshed, and ready to embrace your weight loss journey with confidence, determination, and a profound sense of empowerment."

[Begin the awakening process.]

"1... Starting to awaken now. 2... Feeling more alert. 3... Slowly coming back to your full awareness. 4... Almost there, feeling a sense of empowerment building within you. 5... You are now fully awake, refreshed, and ready to embrace your weight loss journey with enthusiasm and determination."

[End the session with a calm and reassuring tone.]

Chapter 18

Pain Management Script Example

NOTE: Pain can serve an important purpose. Pain should never be removed unless the source of the pain has been identified and removing the pain will not result in further injury.

[After induction and deepener]

"Today, we are going to explore a powerful technique called dissociation to help you manage and reduce your pain. I want you to understand that you have the innate ability to influence your perception of pain and find comfort within yourself."

[Pause, emphasizing the inner strength.]

"Visualize yourself in a serene and peaceful environment. This is your sanctuary, a place where you can experience comfort and tranquility. Picture it in vivid detail, noticing the colors, the gentle sounds, and the soothing sensations."

[Pause as the listener visualizes their sanctuary.]

"As you settle into this sanctuary, imagine a transparent, protective barrier surrounding you. This barrier represents your ability to dissociate from the sensation of pain. It serves as a shield, separating you from the discomfort you are experiencing."

[Pause as the listener envisions the protective barrier.]

"Focus your attention on the area of your body where you are feeling pain. Visualize the pain as a separate entity, like a cloud or a distant object. See it clearly in your mind's eye, separate from your body."

[Pause as the listener dissociates from the pain.]

"Now, imagine the pain slowly drifting away from your body, moving farther and farther away, until it becomes a distant speck in the horizon. Feel the sensation of relief as the pain becomes less and less significant."

[Pause as the listener experiences relief.]

"As the pain continues to move away, notice how the area where you were experiencing discomfort begins to feel lighter and more relaxed. Picture this area bathed in a soothing, healing light, bringing comfort and ease."

[Pause, emphasizing the sensation of relief and comfort.]

"From this moment forward, you have the ability to dissociate from pain whenever it arises. You can visualize it as a separate entity and gently guide it away from your body, finding relief and comfort within yourself."

[Pause, reinforcing the dissociation technique.]

"Whenever you experience pain in the future, you will remember this technique. You can use it to manage and reduce your discomfort, allowing yourself to find comfort and ease even in challenging moments."

[Pause, instilling confidence in the technique.]

"In a moment, I will count from 1 to 5, and with each number, you will become more alert and awake. When I reach the number 5, you will be fully awake, feeling a sense of relief and empowerment."

[Begin the awakening process.]

"1... Starting to awaken now. 2... Feeling more alert. 3... Slowly coming back to your full awareness. 4... Almost there, with a sense of relief. 5... You are now fully awake, feeling a sense of relief and empowerment."

[End the session with a calm and reassuring tone.]

Chapter 19
Anxiety Release Sample Script

[After Induction and depener]

"Today, we are going to work together to help you find a sense c calm and peace within yourself. Understand that you have the inner strength to manage and reduce anxiety. As you continue t relax, know that you are taking an important step towards a more serene and balanced you."

[Pause, emphasizing the inner strength.]

"Visualize yourself in a tranquil and natural setting. This is your sanctuary, a place of serenity and tranquility. Picture it in vivid detail, noticing the colors, the gentle sounds, and the soothing sensations."

[Pause as the listener visualizes their sanctuary.]

"As you immerse yourself in this sanctuary, imagine a warm, healing light enveloping you. This light represents your inner resilience and capacity for relaxation. Feel it wrapping around you, filling you with calmness and tranquility."

[Pause as the listener connects with their inner calm.]

"Now, I want you to become aware of the sensations of anxiety within your body. Notice where you feel it, the physical sensations, and any tension. Visualize the anxiety as a separate entity, like a cloud or a distant object."

[Pause as the listener separates from anxiety.]

"See the anxiety clearly in your mind's eye, detached from your body. Now, imagine the anxiety slowly drifting away from you, moving farther and farther away until it becomes a distant speck in the horizon."

[Pause as the listener experiences anxiety moving away.]

"As the anxiety continues to move away, you feel a profound sense of relief and calmness filling the space it once occupied. Your body and mind become lighter and more relaxed, as if a burden has been lifted."

[Pause as the listener experiences relief.]

"From this moment forward, you have the ability to distance yourself from anxiety whenever it arises. You can visualize it as a separate entity and gently guide it away, allowing yourself to return to a state of calm and tranquility."

[Pause, reinforcing the technique.]

"Whenever anxiety tries to creep in, remember this technique. You can use it to manage and reduce anxiety, finding peace and balance within yourself."

[Pause, instilling confidence in the technique.]

"In a moment, I will count from 1 to 5, and with each number, you will become more alert and awake. When I reach the number 5, you will be fully awake, feeling a sense of calm and inner peace."

[Begin the awakening process.]

"1... Starting to awaken now. 2... Feeling more alert. 3... Slowly coming back to your full awareness. 4... Almost there, with a deep sense of calm. 5... You are now fully awake, feeling calm and at peace."

[End the session with a calm and reassuring tone.]

Chapter 20
Overcoming Fears Sample Script

[After induction and deepener]

"Today, we are going to help you relieve and overcome your fear. I want you to know that you have the inner strength to manage and conquer fear. As you continue to relax, know that you are taking a significant step towards a more fearless you."

[Pause, emphasizing inner strength.]

"Visualize yourself in a beautiful and peaceful movie theater. This theater is your sanctuary, a place where you can experience safety and tranquility. Picture it in vivid detail, noticing the comfortable seats, the serene surroundings, and the soothing ambiance."

[Pause as the listener visualizes the movie theater.]

"As you settle into the theater, imagine a large movie screen in front of you. This screen represents the canvas of your mind, where your fear is currently playing like a movie. You have the power to change the script and the outcome."

[Pause as the listener envisions the movie screen.]

"Picture your fear as a movie on the screen, in full color and motion. See it clearly, but remember that it is just a movie, a creation of your mind. You are safe in the theater, detached from the fear on the screen."

[Pause as the listener observes the fear movie.]

"Now, imagine a remote control in your hand. This remote control allows you to pause, rewind, and change the movie. With confidence, press the pause button, freezing the fear movie on the screen."

[Pause as the listener pauses the fear movie.]

"As you look at the frozen image on the screen, notice that your fear is now a still image, lifeless and powerless. It cannot harm you in this state. Take a deep breath and feel the sense of control and calmness within."

[Pause as the listener experiences control and calmness.]

"Now, use the rewind button on the remote control to rewind the fear movie. See it playing backward at high speed, becoming a blur of images. As it rewinds, notice how it loses its intensity and emotional charge."

[Pause as the listener rewinds the fear movie.]

"Press the play button again, but this time, imagine the fear movie playing in black and white, without sound. See it as a distant and faded memory, no longer holding power over you."

[Pause as the listener watches the faded fear movie.]

"You are in control of the movie. You can choose to stop it, change the script, or simply let it fade into the background. You are the director of your mind's movie theater, and fear no longer has a starring role."

[Pause, emphasizing empowerment.]

"In a moment, I will count from 1 to 5, and with each number, you will become more alert and awake. When I reach the number 5, you will be fully awake, feeling a sense of empowerment and fearlessness."

[Begin the awakening process.]

"1... Starting to awaken now. 2... Feeling more alert. 3... Slowly coming back to your full awareness. 4... Almost there, with a deep sense of empowerment. 5... You are now fully awake, feeling fearless and in control."

[End the session with a calm and reassuring tone.]

Frequently asked questions

Q1: What is hypnosis?

A1: Hypnosis is a natural and altered state of consciousness characterized by focused attention, heightened suggestibility, and deep relaxation. It allows individuals to access their subconscious mind and make positive changes in their thoughts, behaviors, and emotions.

Q2: Is hypnosis the same as being unconscious or asleep?

A2: No, hypnosis is not the same as being unconscious or asleep. In hypnosis, you are fully aware and responsive to suggestions. You are in a highly focused and relaxed state, but you can hear and process information.

Q3: Can anyone be hypnotized?

A3: Yes, anyone can be hypnotized if they allow themselves to be. While the level of hypnotizability varies from person to person, everyone can be hypnotized to some degree. It depends on factors like willingness, belief, and the skill of the hypnotist.

Q4: Is hypnosis safe?

A4: Yes, hypnosis is safe when conducted by a trained and ethical hypnotist. It is a natural state of mind, and you are always in control during a hypnosis session. It cannot make you do anything against your will or values.

Q5: What can hypnosis be used for?

A5: Hypnosis can be used for a wide range of purposes, including stress reduction, anxiety management, pain control, habit change (e.g., quitting smoking or weight loss), improving confidence, and addressing phobias. It is also used in hypnotherapy for various therapeutic goals.

Q6: How long does a hypnosis session last?

A6: The duration of a hypnosis session can vary but typically ranges from 30 minutes to an hour. Some therapeutic sessions may be longer, depending on the goals and needs of the individual.

Q7: Will I remember what happens during a hypnosis session?

A7: Yes, you will generally remember what happens during a hypnosis session. While you may experience deep relaxation and focused attention, you are not in a state of amnesia. You will recall the suggestions and experiences.

Q8: Can I get stuck in hypnosis?

A8: No, you cannot get stuck in hypnosis. You can return to your normal state of consciousness at any time. Hypnosis is a reversible and temporary state.

Q9: Do I have to believe in hypnosis for it to work?

A9: While belief in hypnosis can enhance its effectiveness, it is not a strict requirement. The willingness to follow instructions and the skill of the hypnotist are also important factors.

Q10: Are there any side effects of hypnosis?

A10: Hypnosis is generally considered safe, and side effects are rare. Some individuals may experience minor sensations like drowsiness or slight disorientation after a session, but these are usually temporary.

Q11: Can hypnosis reveal hidden or suppressed memories?

A11: Hypnosis is not a reliable method for uncovering hidden or suppressed memories. Memory recall during hypnosis can be influenced by suggestion, and false memories may be inadvertently created. It is not a substitute for professional therapy in cases of trauma or repressed memories.

Q12: How many sessions are needed for hypnotherapy to be effective?

A12: The number of sessions required for hypnotherapy varies depending on the individual and the specific issue being addressed. Some issues may be resolved in a few sessions, while others may require more extended treatment.

Q13: Can I learn self-hypnosis?

A13: Yes, self-hypnosis is a valuable skill that individuals can learn. It allows you to access the benefits of hypnosis on your own and can be used for self-improvement and relaxation.

Q14: Can hypnosis be done online or through recordings?

A14: Yes, hypnosis can be conducted online or through pre-recorded audio or video sessions. Many individuals find these methods effective for convenience and accessibility. Individual sessions, whether in person or remote over Zoom or similar services are generally more effective as the suggestions can be tailored to your specific needs and issues.

Q15: How do I choose a qualified hypnotist or hypnotherapist?

A15: It's essential to choose a qualified and board-certified hypnotist or hypnotherapist. Consultation and rapport with the therapist are also important factors in your choice.

Remember that while these FAQs provide general information, it's always advisable to consult with a qualified hypnotist or hypnotherapist for personalized guidance and assistance with your specific needs and goals.

Further Reading

"Hypnotherapy: An Exploratory Casebook" by Milton H. Erickson and Ernest L. Rossi - This book offers a collection of case studies by the renowned psychiatrist and hypnotherapist Milton Erickson. It provides valuable insights into the therapeutic applications of hypnosis.

"Trancework: An Introduction to the Practice of Clinical Hypnosis" by Michael D. Yapko - A comprehensive guide to clinical hypnosis, this book covers the fundamentals c hypnotherapy and provides practical techniques for therapists.

"Hypnosis and Hypnotherapy: Basic to Advanced Techniques for the Professional" by Calvin D. Banyan anc Gerald F. Kein - This book is a resource for both beginner and experienced hypnotherapists. It covers a wide range of hypnosis techniques and applications.

"The New Hypnotherapy Handbook: Hypnosis and Mind/Body Healing" by Kevin Hogan - This handbook explores the use of hypnotherapy in mind-body healing, addressing various issues such as pain management, stress reduction, and personal development.

"My Voice Will Go with You: The Teaching Tales of Milton H. Erickson" by Sidney Rosen - A compilation of Milton Erickson's therapeutic stories and metaphors, providing valuable lessons in the use of storytelling in hypnotherapy.

"Handbook of Medical and Psychological Hypnosis: Foundations, Applications, and Professional Issues" edited by Gary Elkins - This comprehensive handbook covers the clinical applications of hypnosis in various medical and psychological fields.

"Hypnotherapy: A Handbook" by Hellmut W. A. Karle and Jennifer H. Boys - An introductory guide to the principles and techniques of hypnotherapy, suitable for both practitioners and those interested in self-hypnosis.

"Foundations of Hypnotherapy: From Mesmer to Freud" by Franz Anton Mesmer, Richard D. Chessick, and David F. Luck - A historical exploration of the foundations of hypnotherapy, tracing its development from Mesmerism to modern hypnosis.

"Hypnosis and Hypnotherapy Patter Scripts and Techniques" by Calvin D. Banyan - A resource for hypnotherapists, this book provides scripts and techniques for various issues, helping practitioners design effective hypnosis sessions.

"The Art of Hypnotherapy" by C. Roy Hunter - This book offers a comprehensive introduction to the art of hypnotherapy, covering techniques, ethics, and case studies.

"Clinical Hypnosis and Self-Regulation: Cognitive-Behavioral Perspectives" by Ursula Havemann-Reinecke and Michael Schmitz - A book that explores the cognitive-behavioral perspective of clinical hypnosis, emphasizing self-regulation and therapeutic applications.

"The Hypnosis Handbook" by Michael Heap - An accessible guide to hypnosis, covering its history, applications, and the science behind it.

"Learn Hypnosis Now" by Michael Stevenson - This book by Michael Stevenson provides practical insights and techniques for learning hypnosis.

"Crushing Cancer...Now" by Tim Moore - This book contains valuable information related to incorporating th mind in overcoming cancer treatment symptoms and side effects.

These references and books offer a comprehensive understanding of hypnosis and its applications, from therapeutic use to self-improvement. Depending on your specific interests, you can explore these resources to gain knowledge in the field of hypnosis.

About The Author

Tim Moore is a Board Certified Clinical Hypnotherapist, Certified Master Hypnotherapist, and Master NLP Practitioner and Hypnotherapy Trainer. Tim believes in a compassionate therapy approach focused on the mind-body connection. He has been student of the mind for nearly 30 years, exploring it's inner workings. He is also a member of various international hypnotherapy and coaching boards. Tim's work is centered on helping clients achieve health and wellness through powerful mind-directed techniques.

Tim grew up an introvert, but once learning how to use the subconscious mind was able to reprogram himself and change from introvert to being able to become a public speaker, author and leading clinical Hypnotherapist.

For more information on Tim, you can visit
www.mindoverthebody.com

For more information on becoming a certified Hypnotherapist, visit the Hypno-Mastery Training Page at
www.hypno-mastery.com

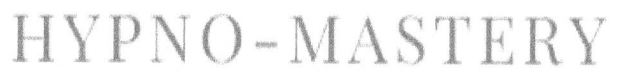

HYPNO-MASTERY

HYPNOTHERAPY TRAINING & CERTIFICATION